Pocket Guide to Teaching for Clinical Instructors

Previously known as *Pocket Guide to Teaching for Medical Instructors* with the new emphasis acknowledging the broader target audience and community of interest

Pocket Guide to Teaching for Clinical Instructors

Third Edition

Advanced Life Support Group and Resuscitation Council (UK)

Edited by

Ian Bullock

London, Executive Director, Care Quality Improvement Department
COO, National Clinical Guideline Centre, Royal College of Physicians
Lead Educator, RC(UK), GIC Working Group

Mike Davis

Blackpool, Consultant in Continuing Medical Education
Lead Educator, ALSG, GIC Working Group

Andrew Lockey

Halifax, Consultant in Emergency Medicine
Director of Medical Education, Calderdale and Huddersfield Foundation Trust
Clinical Lead, RC(UK), GIC Working Group

Kevin Mackway-Jones

Manchester, Consultant in Emergency Medicine, Central Manchester Foundation Trust
Medical Director, North West Ambulance Service
Clinical Lead, ALSG, GIC Working Group

WILEY Blackwell   BMJ|Books

This edition first published 2016 © 2016 by John Wiley & Sons, Ltd

First edition © 1998 by BMJ Books; Second edition © 2008 by Blackwell Publishing.

BMJ Books is an imprint of BMJ Publishing Group Limited, used under licence by John Wiley & Sons.

Registered office: John Wiley & Sons, Ltd, The Atrium, Southern Gate, Chichester, West Sussex, PO19 8SQ, UK

Editorial offices: 9600 Garsington Road, Oxford, OX4 2DQ, UK
The Atrium, Southern Gate, Chichester, West Sussex, PO19 8SQ, UK
1606 Golden Aspen Drive, Suites 103 and 104, Ames, Iowa 50010, USA

For details of our global editorial offices, for customer services and for information about how to apply for permission to reuse the copyright material in this book please see our website at www.wiley.com/wiley-blackwell

Library of Congress Cataloging-in-Publication Data

Pocket guide to teaching for clinical instructors / Advanced Life Support Group and Resuscitation Council (UK) ; edited by Ian Bullock, Mike Davis, Andrew Lockey, and Kevin Mackway-Jones. – Third edition.
   p. ; cm.
   Includes bibliographical references and index.
   ISBN 978-1-118-86007-6 (pbk.)
   I. Bullock, Ian, editor.   II. Davis, Mike, 1947- , editor.   III. Lockey, Andrew, editor.
IV. Mackway-Jones, Kevin, editor.   V. Advanced Life Support Group (Manchester, England), issuing body.   VI. Resuscitation Council (UK), issuing body.
   [DNLM: 1. Teaching–methods. 2. Health Personnel–education. W 18]
   R833.5
   610.71'1–dc23   2015004894

A catalogue record for this book is available from the British Library.

Wiley also publishes its books in a variety of electronic formats. Some content that appears in print may not be available in electronic books.

Set in 10/12pt PalatinoLTStd by Aptara Inc., New Delhi, India
Printed and bound in Malaysia by Vivar Printing Sdn Bhd

2   2016

Contents

Working group

Ian Bullock
London

Mike Davis
Blackpool

Sue Hampshire
London

Andrew Lockey
Halifax

Kevin Mackway-Jones
Manchester

Sarah Mitchell
London

Sue Wieteska
Manchester

Contributors to the third edition

Ian Bullock
London

Mike Davis
Blackpool

Kate Denning
Plymouth

Sue Hampshire
London

Andrew Lockey
Halifax

Kevin Mackie
Birmingham

Kevin Mackway-Jones
Manchester

Sarah Mitchell
London

Elizabeth Norris
Bath

Sue Wieteska
Manchester

Contributors to the first and second editions

Ian Bullock
London

Andrew Coleman
Northampton

Mick Colquhoun
Cardiff

Pat Conaghan
Manchester

Mike Davis
Blackpool

Kate Denning
Plymouth

Peter Driscoll
Manchester

David Gabbott
Bristol

Carl Gwinnutt
Manchester

Bob Harris
London

Duncan Harris
London

Sara Harris
London

Jane Hatfield
Oxford

Gareth Holsgrove
Cambridge

Pauline Howard
Oxford

Melanie Humphreys
Wolverhampton

Lynn Jones
Manchester

Andrew Lockey
Halifax

Kevin Mackie
Birmingham

Kevin Mackway-Jones
Manchester

Sarah Mitchell
London

Jerry Nolan
Oxford

Gavin Perkins
Birmingham

Russell Perkins
Manchester

Mike Walker
London

Terence Wardle
Chester

Celia Warlow
Northampton

Sue Wieteska
Manchester

Jonathan Wyllie
Middlesbrough

Jackie Younker
Bristol

Foreword

The third edition of the *Pocket Guide to Teaching for Clinical Instructors* (commonly known as the 'Blue Book') is certainly a success story. Written for the first time in 1998 by medical educators engaged with the RC (UK) and the ALSG to support the generic instructor courses (GIC), it was quickly appreciated throughout Europe with its second expanded edition published in 2008. Translations into several languages followed and during the last few years it was adopted by the ERC as the written teaching source for their GIC.

Some might argue that teaching is a practical skill that ignites the learning process and it cannot be learnt from a book. Without solid theoretical background about how learning is promoted through different teaching approaches, a medical instructor's entire teaching effort is reduced to empiricism and merely passing on beliefs.

It is fascinating how the authors of the 'blue book', all excellent practitioners in teaching, have been able to condense their knowledge into the well-structured chapters of this book. As a guide for instructors, it is not just another textbook on teaching in medicine.

It is a comprehensive and concise theoretical framework for effective teaching in life support courses and contains many practical tips. Reading this book before or after a GIC helps one to understand the background of the discussions and exercises, and gain keen insight into how teaching can be improved.

New chapters have been added to this new edition, which reflects the current developments of the learning needs in the GIC. Scenario teaching and role play are now discussed under the title of simulation. Instructors are not only expected to 'run a scenario', but rather to try as much as possible to imitate the clinical reality of the course candidates. This connects the learning objectives of the simulation to the daily clinical practice of the participants with the aim of fostering deeper understanding and enhancing retention. Important background is provided on how to 'buy in' professionals even in low and very low fidelity simulation settings, which is the case in many resuscitation courses.

Other important adaptations include the 'learning conversation' as a more direct approach to feedback. It's a move away from a rather closed structure of feedback as in the 'feedback sandwich' or also the Pendleton model of feedback. The learning conversation opens a discussion about the views of the participants on events during simulation and includes other team members in critical reflection with the instructor. All this is funnelled down in the end to an action plan for new learning goals to improve performance.

In the last few years, the patient safety movement has recommended that increasing attention should be given to non-technical skills (NTS) in medicine. Therefore, this version of the book encourages instructors to also teach NTS during life support courses. The reader will find a chapter on the teaching of teams, which touches upon differences between teaching individuals and groups and what makes an effective working team. That is of utmost importance for the challenges medicine faces in the 21st century.

The chapter 'Supporting Learners' takes up the team teaching idea and adds to the discussion about the 'role of the instructor' with important perspectives on mentoring candidates. This chapter also includes new inputs on the function and purpose of faculty meetings and how they can improve teaching and learning in GIC.

I hope this edition will meet the expectations of medical instructors and help them to improve their teaching so that the newest medical knowledge can to be translated into effective inter-professional and inter-disciplinary team-based patient treatment.

Robert Tino Greif
Director of Training and Education, European Resuscitation Council
Bern, Switzerland

This concise but comprehensive publication (the so called 'blue-book') will provide background reading for participants and instructors before and after their ERC GIC. With this support, the ERC and ALSG/RC (UK) authors and editors wish all GIC-participants successful teaching experiences on their provider courses.

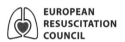

**EUROPEAN
RESUSCITATION
COUNCIL**

Preface to the third edition

It is with great pleasure that we introduce the third edition of the "Blue Book" to you. Our first edition in 1998 laid some important foundations for the practice of course presentation and reflection on that experience; our second edition in 2008 built on these and extended the original approach in breadth and depth. This latest edition reflects ongoing developments and adaptations, including the introduction of blended learning in instructor training and the nature of the changing role of the instructors, particularly in relation to giving feedback, the structure and purpose of small group teaching and further thoughts on initiating and maintaining psychological realism in simulated learning events. We introduce for the first time, attention to non-technical skills and a focus on management of life support being a team, as opposed to an individual, endeavour.

We continue to provide a firm basis for the more practical components by drawing attention to important and relevant adult education theory. We also continue to maintain a robust model of effective planning and preparation for the variety of teaching modalities that you are likely to meet on courses. We recognise the contribution that this can make to other teaching that you might engage in your day to day interaction with colleagues and elsewhere.

We welcome the endorsement of the European Resuscitation Council and its formal adoption of the Blue Book as background reading for their instructors and candidates on their Generic Instructor Course.

The Blue Book is now just one element of a more complex educational experience than that which emerged in the late 20th century. While some elements remain the same such as a commitment to sound practices in adult learning others have had to respond to, sometimes competing, pressures. Blended learning is now a key ingredient of much of medical and other health care related courses at undergraduate level and continuing medical education has to reflect that change in practices. Nevertheless, there is still the need for a small, portable and well written book: hence the new edition of the *Pocket Guide to Teaching for Clinical Instructors*. We hope you enjoy it.

Ian Bullock
Mike Davis
Andrew Lockey
Kevin Mackway-Jones
(Editors)

Preface to the first edition

This short guide is in two parts. Part one begins by introducing the basic principles under teaching and then goes on to deal in more detail with a number of modes of teaching on courses. Lectures skill stations, scenarios, workshops and discussions are dealt with here. In each case practical guidance is given to help the reader to become a more effective teacher.

Part two covers many of the same areas again, but this time giving more background information and describing some more advanced instructional skills. It deals with the nature of adult learning, the four domains of learning, the learning process, questions and answers, role play, mentoring and problems with workshops and discussions. Each topic is presented as a short section which can be sampled to help with specific issues.

The guide is intended as an aid to reflection: something which you can, and hopefully will, consult on many occasions before, during and after your courses. It does not contain all the answers, but it will at least provide an alternative voice, something to argue with and something against which you can test your experiences. This guide does not attempt to provide a blueprint for teaching, rather it gives advice about the basics which once mastered will be adapted to your personality and creativity. In the end, of course, it is what works for you that matters.

In the long run it does not matter greatly whether you read this guide before or after a course (although most courses will require you to read beforehand). Knowledge and skill as a teacher build up gradually, provided you are able to reflect upon your teaching experiences and continue to learn.

Good luck with your teaching.

Mike Walker
Kevin Mackway-Jones
(Editorial Board)

Acknowledgments

A great many people have put a lot of hard work into the production of this book, and the accompanying generic instructor course. The editors would like to thank all the contributors for their efforts.

Finally, we would like to thank, in advance, those of you who will engage with all aspects of the GIC (this book, the VLE, the face to face course and the instructor candidacies); no doubt you will have lots of constructive criticism to offer.

CHAPTER 1

Adult learning

Learning outcomes

By the end of this chapter you should be able to demonstrate an understanding of
- how adults learn
- the contribution of experiential learning
- motivation

Introduction

While adult learners differ from children and adolescents in a wide variety of ways (largely as a consequence of the voluntary character of adult learning), they retain some characteristics, particularly a perceived need to see the teacher as a fount of all knowledge and insight. In general, however, adult learners (and health professionals in particular) can be thought of as having the capacity to demonstrate different attributes (Knowles, 1973).

Knowles and the adult learner

Autonomy and self-determination
These are not always possible in formal learning but, in general, health professionals have at least the capacity to take decisions about the direction and timing of their learning. This aspect is particularly important when engaging with blended learning environments comprising virtual learning environment (VLE) and face-to-face experiences. Where decisions are taken out of their hands – for example by being sent on a course – there may be some initial resistance unless learning can be experienced as stimulating

Pocket Guide to Teaching for Clinical Instructors, Third Edition.
Edited by Ian Bullock, Mike Davis, Andrew Lockey and Kevin Mackway-Jones.
© 2016 John Wiley & Sons, Ltd. Published 2016 by John Wiley & Sons, Ltd.

and valuable. This clearly has implications for motivation and this will be explored later in the chapter.

Life experience and knowledge

Most health professionals have had many years of formal full-time education (13 years in school, 3–6 years in higher education) and many more years in postgraduate training. No matter how receptive they may be to new ideas, there is a great deal of conservatism which needs to be overcome before learning can occur. This has been represented by Lewin (1951) in the following way:

Unfreezing – change – refreezing
Unfreezing is the point at which the learner becomes open to the idea of change (in understanding, affect, skill level); change is then incorporated and reinforced through feedback and ongoing practice both in the training environment and in the workplace.

Goal orientated
Many adults like to have an outcome or a clear product from their efforts. Learning for its own sake may have some attractions at certain times, but it is not a luxury that busy professionals can include in their working lives.

Relevance orientated
Similarly, learning has to be relevant to work-based practices if it is to be valued by learners. As well as subject matter, this also relates to level: material can fail to be relevant if it is too easy or too complex. Content needs to be constructed around the experiences of the learner. In this case, the learning is located quite explicitly within a 'community of practice' and this will be explored later in the chapter.

Practical
Learners get a great deal from integrating skills, knowledge and affect in complex, practical learning events, preferably related to previous experience and/or expectation of future practice. Nana Gitz Holler (Denmark), a learner on a European Provider Course, wrote

> ... we are not machines and this course gives room for us to think and makes the whole teaching session and the teamwork alive and interesting. It opens up for discussions and that is where you really learn something – not only from the instructors but also from the other candidates.

Esteem

Ask health professionals about negative experiences of learning and they are likely to mention humiliation. Good education acknowledges the contribution that learners can make to the learning of others including the teachers (and respects their achievements thus far).

The experiential learning cycle

There are a number of theories of adult learning that are relevant to those involved in continuing medical education, but it is beyond the scope of this book to explore them all. Relevant titles are included in the references at the end of each chapter for those who are interested in exploring some of these. However, there is one theory that is useful to explore briefly here, that of experiential learning.

This theory was based on ideas about reflection developed in the 1930s by John Dewey (1938). One of the components is the experiential learning cycle, illustrated in Figure 1.1.

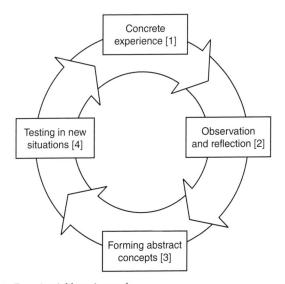

Figure 1.1 Experiential learning cycle

Source: Kolb 1975. Reprinted with permission of Wiley & Sons.

This model, attributed to Kolb and Fry (1975), is a helpful source of explanation for what we do all the time. We have hundreds of experiences every day, but most of them pass us by. If, however, we are to learn from them, we have to be willing and able to go round the cycle.

Experience, any event, however small. Enabling learners to utilise experience provides the foundation for them to maximise learning.

Observation and reflection is the process of describing the event and trying to understand its significance. This stage can sometimes be captured by asking the following questions:

- What happened?
- What did it feel like?

These questions are intended to enable the learner to look in some detail at events and identify some of their emotional components.

Forming abstract concepts is an attempt to generalise from the specific, by asking:

- What does it mean?
- Do I need to change?

Take as an example, being late for a workshop. The focus of your observation and reflection will (inevitably) be related to that specific event, that is being late on that occasion and your thinking might be: 'The next time I am due to lead a workshop, I will set off a little earlier'. The conceptualisation phase, however, will explore being late in other contexts and the generalisation would be framed in more general terms, thus: 'When I am due to go somewhere to do something, I will set off earlier than I think I need to, just in case something holds me up on the way'. This kind of thinking therefore leads into

Testing in new situations, considering the question:

- How might I be different in the future?

Note that it is 'I' being different. It is easier to change your own behaviour than it is to change that of others.

By going round the experiential learning cycle, a learner can capitalise on personal insight into events that are often taken for granted, but which can benefit from closer examination. Most experiences probably do not justify this exploration, but if behaviour seems to be working against us (e.g. as in the case of being habitually late), there is some real merit in exploring experience in a more systematic way.

In the context of continuing medical education, the experiential learning cycle has the merit of the systematic, shared exploration of repeat practice in a controlled environment, with feedback and discussion seeking to achieve improvement and develop competence which can be employed back in the workplace (see Chapter 8).

Blended learning

As is explored in Chapter 9, technology has had an impact on the nature of the learning environment and the way in which the learning experience is structured. A number of myths exist about e-learning and can often misinform the learner even before they access a VLE. Mattheos et al. (2001) describe these myths as

a passing fad, only for knowledge acquisition, ineffective and inefficient, loneliness in learning, redundant teachers, technology predominating and it being an unrealistic dream.

This need not be the case. A flexible blended learning opportunity can be at least equivalent or better than traditional face-to-face teaching. For adult learners, there are significant advantages, with relevant content, wide choice and supportive guidance enabling them to choose when they learn, in proximity to additional training/learning or the frequency of learning. As a strategy, it encourages reflection on and in learning, developing these transferable skills into other learning settings, such as simulated practice or group discussion.

The success of blended learning implementation is well demonstrated in the paper evaluating the implementation of the eALS (Perkins et al., 2012). Another paper (Thorne CJ et al., 2015) provides further evidence of the positive impact of blended learning environments.

Situated learning

Situated learning (Lave and Wenger, 1991) is particularly important for adult learners, especially in the context of continuing education, in that it acknowledges the existence of working lives. In the case of doctors and other health professionals, much learning relates directly to their day-to-day practices and as such can be seen as being a component of their situation. Among the features of situated learning is the notion of the community of practice and it is this that will now be explored.

Community of practice

Communities of practice stem from the notion of shared experience and ways of thinking and talking about that experience. Consider the word 'shock'. What it means to an ED doctor or a paramedic is different to the meaning ascribed to it when someone is describing a surprising social encounter. This crude example is multiplied by the subtleties in language use and other behaviour that can derive from exposure a group of people going about their professional lives.

A way of exploring this is to invite you to reflect on your experience of taking up a new post. There are a number of things you have to come to terms with

- This is what we do
- The patients always have their tea before the ward round
- The Prof always comes in on Thursdays
- That is Bob's chair/cup/computer
- Did we tell you about the time when …

In translating these behaviours into the structures associated with a community of practice we can see the following:

Practices	This is what we do
Routines	The patients always have their tea before the ward round
Rituals	The Prof always comes in on Thursdays
Artefacts/symbols	That is Bob's chair/cup/computer
Stories and histories	Did we tell you about the time when…

Until you become familiar with some or all of these (and their close and distant relations), you are a newcomer and capable of getting some things wrong, or at least 'Not the way we do it here'. As such, you are a participant, but not a full participant: situated learning describes your status as that of 'legitimate, peripheral participation'. Depending on the force of your personality, and/or your capacity for compliance, it may not be long before you become a full member of the community of practice and it, in turn, may have altered its behaviour slightly in acknowledgment of your impact.

Significant informal learning takes place within the community of practice. Its relevance for courses wanting to contribute towards effective professional performance is that the informal, temporary communities that they create should be similar to those from which the learners come. This is particularly important when setting up and running simulations which, while not being able to replicate 'real life' fully in terms of equipment and human patients, should aspire towards a psychological realism that reflects what people might find in their own practice.

Maximising motivation

Adult learners have to be motivated if they are going to learn and the principle of voluntarism is a key feature of successful adult learning experiences. Almost by definition, learners in continual medical education contexts will be voluntary – in that nobody is forcing them to attend a programme. Nevertheless, they may be extrinsically motivated, that is the factors that are influencing their attendance may be driven by outside forces. In the context of continuing medical education these include gaining recognition, having something to put on a CV or filling a need for career progression.

Malone and Lepper (1987) have detailed how intrinsic motivation has different, and predominantly internal, drivers and these can be summarised as in Table 1.1.

Table 1.1 Intrinsic motivation

Factors	Elements
Challenge	Meaningful goals that challenge learners just beyond their comfort zones
Curiosity	An expectation that there may be better ways of doing things; that there are things that you do not know
Independence	Learners demonstrating the need to move towards autonomy
Imagination	The capacity to work in 'let's pretend' environments (see particularly Chapter 5) where risks can be taken in safety
Social comparison	The desire to judge personal performance against that of others
Interdependence	The willingness to contribute towards others' learning
Esteem	Knowing that success will contribute towards feeling good about oneself

Extrinsic motivation is often regarded as 'bad' in comparison to 'good' intrinsic motivation, and it is generally true that people are more likely to own up to intrinsic drivers when asked, for example, why they are attending a course. It is likely that most individuals are motivated both extrinsically and intrinsically. Those motivated solely by external factors can, however, still be effective learners if certain needs are met.

Most reports of Maslow's hierarchy of needs (1971) have five layers in the pyramid, but the model shown in Figure 1.2 acknowledges his later thinking.

This classical theory of motivation demands that much of the lower-level needs have to be met before the learner can move up to the next level. In practical terms, this means that an educational experience has to guarantee a number of conditions. These are explored in Table 1.2.

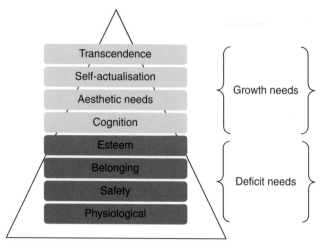

Figure 1.2 Maslow's hierarchy of needs (http://chiron.valdosta.edu/whuitt/COL/motivation/motivate.html)

Source: Adapted from Huitt 2011.

Table 1.2 Maslow's hierarchy of needs

Need	Implications for programme design and presentation
Physiological needs (to maintain homeostasis)	
Warmth, food, drink, shelter, sex	Attention to the environment: adequate accommodation, regular refreshment breaks, a reasonable working day
Safety needs (to be free from the threat of aggression, hostility)	
Physical and psychological security	Guaranteeing freedom from external threats (fire, etc.); secure boundaries; no obvious ego threat
Social needs (to develop a sense of belonging)	
Legitimate membership; community	The opportunity to interact through social exchange (e.g. during registration, but also in opening activities through introductions and an opportunity to share experiences, thinking)
Esteem needs (to develop a sense of self-worth and the capacity to engender that in others	
Respect, confidence, competence	The opportunity to acquire knowledge and skills and the ability to manifest appropriate attitudes through structured learning interventions with supportive and authentic feedback

Table 1.2 Maslow's hierarchy of needs (*Continued*)

Need	Implications for programme design and presentation
Cognitive needs (to know and understand)	
Different levels of cognition:	Through demonstration, modelling, specific instruction and feedback, learners can move through the levels via:
• Knowledge	
• Comprehension	Cognition: types of questions
• Application	Skills: four-stage approach
• Analysis	Attitudes: encouragement appropriate affect
• Synthesis	(e.g. team membership)
• Evaluation	
Different levels of skill acquisition	
• Perception	
• Guided response	
• Mastery	
• Autonomy	
Different levels of attitudes	
• Perceiving	
• Complying	
• Accepting	
• Internalising	
Aesthetic needs (to value symmetry, order)	
	A programme that works, e.g. runs to time, experienced and competent instructors who care about learning – for themselves and others – and fun
Self-actualisation (to be an autonomous individual)	
In touch with reality	An experienced faculty capable of manifesting these
Acceptance of self and others	behaviours as a matter of routine gives learners confidence and also models appropriate behaviour
Spontaneous	
Problem-solving	
Tolerance of ambiguity	
Gemeinschaftsgefühl (empathy and compassion)	
Creativity	
Self-transcendence (to develop actualisation among others)	
Concern for others' development	As above
Ego security – not threatened by others' achievements	

Maslow's theory has been criticised for its lack of scientific rigour, but it does have some useful things to say about how events can be organised and presented. It is certainly true that unless the basic needs at the bottom of the hierarchy are met, at least to some extent, then learning will be hampered. Accordingly, attention to the conditions within which learning is to take place is essential. More important, however, is the psychological domain within which people will interact with others in a complex, dynamic environment. It is the responsibility of the trainer to ensure that this is a challenging but safe area within which people will learn.

Summary and learning

Adults are usually voluntary learners and need to be actively engaged in their own learning. They need goal-orientated, relevant, practical experiences in order to get the most from teaching. Where possible, this should have its origins in the workplace environments from which learners come. While many admit only to intrinsic motivation the reality is that many external factors affect this as well. Blended learning opportunities offer adult learners both variety and enable choices to be made regarding when and how they learn.

References

Dewey J. *Experience and Education*. Collier Books, New York, 1938.

Knowles M. *The Adult Learner: A Neglected Species*. Gulf Publishing, Houston, 1973.

Kolb DA, Fry R. Toward an applied theory of experiential learning. In: Cooper C, ed. *Theories of Group Process*. John Wiley, London, 1975.

Lave J, Wenger E. *Situated Learning: Legitimate Peripheral Participation*. University of Cambridge Press, Cambridge, 1991

Lewin K. *Field Theory in Social Science: Selected Theoretical Papers*. Harper & Row, New York, 1951.

Malone TW, Lepper MR. Making learning fun: a taxonomy of intrinsic motivations for learning. In: Snow RE, Farr MJ, eds. *Aptitude, Learning and Instruction: III. Cognitive and Affective Process Analyses*. Erlbaum, Hillsdale, NJ, 1987.

Maslow A. *The Farther Reaches of Human Nature*. The Viking Press, New York, 1971. http://chiron.valdosta.edu/whuitt/COL/motivation/motivate.html

Mattheos N, Nattestad A, Schittek M, Attstrom R. A virtual classroom for undergraduate periodontology: a pilot study. *European Journal of Dental Education*, 2001;5:139–147.

Perkins GD, Bullock I, Clutton-Brock T, Davies RP, Gale M, Lam J, Lockey A, Kimani PK, Stallard N. Blended advanced life support training: a multi-country randomised controlled non-inferiority trial. *Ann Intern Med*, 2012;157(1):19–28.

Thorne CJ, Lockey AS, Bullock I, Hampshire S, Begum-Ali S, Perkins GD. e-Learning in Advanced Life Support – An Evaluation by the Resuscitation Council UK. *Resuscitation*, 2015;90:79–84.

CHAPTER 2

A structured approach to teaching

Learning outcomes

By the end of this chapter you should be able to demonstrate an understanding of the structured approach to teaching, specifically
- Environment
- Set
- Dialogue
- Closure

Introduction

This chapter sets out the basic principles of teaching which will be used throughout the guide. These principles can be used to plan and present all forms of teaching, whether lectures, discussions, workshops, skill stations or simulations.

Teaching may be defined as a *planned experience which brings about a change in behaviour*. The important words here are 'planned' and 'change in behaviour'. We all learn from experience, but teaching involves a planned intention to bring about the learning of specified material which will result in a desired outcome.

There are always four stages to consider: these are discussed in more detail below.

Environment

The teaching environment is an integral part of the teaching process. All aspects of the environment should be considered.

Pocket Guide to Teaching for Clinical Instructors, Third Edition.
Edited by Ian Bullock, Mike Davis, Andrew Lockey and Kevin Mackway-Jones.
© 2016 John Wiley & Sons, Ltd. Published 2016 by John Wiley & Sons, Ltd.

These include heating, lighting, ventilation, acoustics and the arrangement of the furniture. By addressing these issues, you are meeting the physiological needs identified by Maslow (1987) and explored in chapter 1.

The environment can radically affect how a teaching session is conducted and how it will be received by the learners. For example, rows of chairs restrict participation, whereas a circle implies that everyone is expected to contribute. Suboptimal heating and lighting can undermine a teaching session which has otherwise been meticulously prepared. Students who cannot hear the instructor or see a demonstration will find it difficult to achieve the learning outcomes.

The environment must be conducive to the learning that has been planned.

Set

Set is about creating the conditions within which learning can be maximised. It has been described in a number of ways but the essential components need to include

- Atmosphere
- Motivation
- Outcomes
- Roles

These are 'set' in the first few minutes of any session. It is during this time that the instructor will establish the *atmosphere* suggested by the environment and enhance the learners' *motivation* by demonstrating the usefulness of the content for them. During set, the *learning outcomes* will be stated, outlining the territory to be explored. The learners' and instructor's *roles* will be made clear, for example the learners should be told about the nature and extent of their engagement – if they are going to be asked questions, engage in buzz-group activities, be observers, etc.

Practically, they need to know who you are, who they are and what they are going to do during your session. It will be best to avoid telling them that 'This is the most important lecture you are going to hear today' if only to avoid upsetting your colleagues who are to follow. However, it is worth spelling out the significance of the session and how it fits into the programme as a whole. A statement of objectives or learning outcomes provides a useful agenda for the session and gives you something to return to during the final part of the session. Your audience need to have a sense of what their role might be: let them know if you are going to ask them questions or engage in discussions with others. Tell them if you are willing to take questions during the session or reserve questions for the end. A purposeful atmosphere is rarely achieved by telling a joke. Set prepares the group for learning.

Dialogue

This is the main part of the planned experience and involves an interaction between learner and teacher that brings about the planned change in behaviour. Dialogue contains the essential subject matter, whether it be a lecture, workshop, discussion or simulation. This represents the central core of the session and will be by far the longest section.

There are many ways of conducting the dialogue depending on the teaching modality. Irrespective of the technique used, the instructor must ensure that the content is available to the learner in a clear and logical form, and at a level which can be understood. This will be explored in more detail in each of the chapters dealing with the different modalities.

Checking whether the ideas have been understood usually involves questions and answers in one form or another. Giving an appropriate response to the learner's question or comment – a response that promotes learning – is an important element of the dialogue.

Closure

The final part of the teaching session should be the closure. A teaching session, which does not end clearly but just drifts to an end, not only has an unsatisfactory feel about it, but may also leave unanswered questions in the students' mind. A good closure has three parts:
• Questions
• Summary
• Termination
A period for questions from the students allows any remaining problems to be aired and dealt with. A concise summary revisits the learning outcomes from set, pulls together the key points of the session and relates them to other parts of the course or programme of study. Finally, the termination ends the session. The latter can be achieved in a variety of ways. The most obvious is direct verbal instruction linked with a break in eye contact and a physical move away from the class.

In the chapters which follow you will find that each mode of teaching is broken down into the four constituent phases – environment, set, dialogue and closure as discussed above.

Summary and learning

A structured approach can be applied to all teaching interventions. By ensuring that attention is paid to the environment, the set is clear, the dialogue is engaging and the closure is appropriate, the learning experience will be optimised.

Reference

Maslow A. *Motivation and Personality*, 3rd ed. Harper & Row, New York, 1987.

CHAPTER 3
Lecturing effectively

Learning outcomes

By the end of this chapter you should be able to demonstrate an understanding of
- the value of the lecture
- the importance of questions
- what and how you communicate

Introduction

The lecture is a relatively low-risk educational tool that enables a message to be reliably conveyed to an audience. At its best, the lecture is a means of transmitting knowledge in a standardised format. At its worst, it is based on a culture of silence – lectures traditionally can be seen and experienced as passive events. It has even been said that a lecture is a process by which the notes of the lecturer become the notes of the student without passing through the mind of either. There is some truth in that. There is, however, a considerable body of evidence that active learning is required if adult learners are going to benefit from an educational intervention. This chapter will explore ways in which a lecture can be interactive, and thereby a more powerful experience for both teacher and learners in order to reach its potential as a learning experience.

The benefits of lectures are usually summarised as follows:
- Disseminating information (possibly to large numbers)
- Reducing the risk of ambiguity
- Stimulating learner interest

Pocket Guide to Teaching for Clinical Instructors, Third Edition.
Edited by Ian Bullock, Mike Davis, Andrew Lockey and Kevin Mackway-Jones.
© 2016 John Wiley & Sons, Ltd. Published 2016 by John Wiley & Sons, Ltd.

- Introducing learners to content/tasks before other instructional processes

Disseminating information

The lecture enables specific messages to be conveyed to an audience. The advent of web-based presentations has meant that lectures can be simultaneously watched by millions of viewers, either live or pre-recorded. More commonly in continuing medical education, your audience is likely to be relatively small (12–30). Nevertheless, it is an opportunity to give the same message to a whole group of learners. This does not, of course, mean that the same message has been *received* by all the individuals in the room.

Reducing ambiguity

Lectures rarely break new ground, they are much more likely to provide the opportunity to clarify information that students have learned in other contexts – for example reading a text or watching a demonstration. Questions, in both directions, can contribute to this process.

Stimulating learner interest

When you ask people to recall the best lecture they have ever heard, they are more likely to comment on the personal style, charisma and entertainment value of the lecturer rather than its content. What lecturers are doing in these cases is encouraging, albeit subtly, their audience to go away and do some reading and thinking about their subject matter.

Introducing content

Lectures can, therefore, lay the foundations for more detailed study by signposting learners in particular directions.

Lectures do have a number of limitations, including the inability to teach skills. It is also difficult to present complex and/or particularly abstract ideas. However, the main disadvantage is one of learner attention span. This varies considerably among learners with reports ranging from 10 minutes upwards. It all depends on a variety of factors – particularly levels of engagement.

As shown in Chapter 2, a structure (environment, set, dialogue and closure) can be applied to any teaching session. Lectures are no exception.

Environment

It is important to check your environment before you are due to give your lecture. It is a good idea, therefore, to arrive in plenty of time before you are due to talk. You should then

- *Check the layout*: It is likely that a room will be set up for a lecture (i.e. rows of chairs facing a screen) but someone may have been running a workshop before you, and chairs may be in a circle or horseshoe.
- *Test the projection facilities*: In most cases, you will find a computer and data projector but make sure you are familiar with the computer, where to put your flash drive, or whether there is a remote control. For peace of mind, have a backup for your presentation. One way of doing this is to email your presentation to yourself and/or the local organiser or have it available on cloud-based storage.
- *Adjust temperature and lighting*: If the room has been occupied for some time, open windows or run the air conditioning; make sure that your slides are visible with lights on or dimmed.
- *Check for a clock*: If there is not one visible, remind yourself to use your watch. Contrary to opinion, it is not distracting for a lecturer to keep an eye on the time.

Set

Your slides should include learning outcomes or objectives. These serve a number of purposes, including giving your audience a sense of where your session is going. The set is the opportunity you have to claim credibility, by virtue of who you are and what you do. The audience will already have made an assessment of you based on your appearance, but they need to be reassured that you are qualified to be introducing the topic to them. It is not immodest to lay claim to your professional role and your expertise in a particular area. You do, of course, have to live up to the claims you make by being authoritative and knowledgeable. This might include owning up to not knowing something when asked a question. Your claim to credibility can be reinforced by checking with faculty colleagues in the audience or saying that you will find the answer to a question and letting people know. That is preferable to making something up, guessing or giving a partial answer.

During the set it is useful to let your audience know what roles they will be expected to fill: whether they can ask questions for instance or whether you will be asking them to engage in any activities. You might like to let them know if you are going to give them handouts or make your presentation available to them electronically. This will determine whether or not they wish to take notes.

Unlike in a wedding speech, you are not required to tell jokes. Unless you have good comic timing and your jokes are appropriate and funny, this can be a high-risk strategy.

Dialogue

Put quite simply, the dialogue is the content and the substance of the learning outcomes you introduced in the set. In some cases, you will be working from pre-prepared slide sets, which have an approved content. In other cases, you will be presenting your own slides. Whatever the situation, much of the experience for the audience will be in how you present your information, rather that the information itself. In fact, some experts argue that only 7% of communication is about the words you speak, as Figure 3.1 suggests. This raises some important issues when considering the components of what makes a successful presentation.

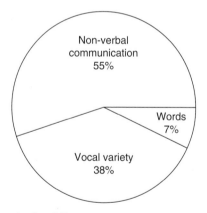

Figure 3.1 Communication skills

Vocal variety
Vocal variety or verbal style refers to
- Voice
- Emphasis

- Pace
- Enthusiasm

You might think that there is nothing you can do about your voice, but that is not entirely the case. Pitch and projection are two things that will ensure that your audience can hear you. Certain sections may need emphasis and you will develop a personal style as to how this can be achieved. Strategies range from slowing down, repetition and simply telling the audience what you are going to say. The pace at which you speak is important even when you are not expecting your audience to take notes. Slightly slower than normal conversation gives your audience time to reflect on what you are saying. Enthusiasm is very contagious as unfortunately is its opposite. Generally, you should communicate your interest in your subject by speaking about it with a degree of animation. Manic fervour may, however, distract the audience from the content.

Verbal tics can become a distraction to an audience, who focus on how many times you use a word or phrase rather than listening to the content. Common ones are 'OK', 'so ... ', 'you know' or 'umm'. Linguists call these 'hesitation phenomena', and they are a product of either lack of confidence or working memory capacity. More often than not, speakers are not aware of their tics so it is advisable to get feedback from colleagues.

Non-verbal communication

Those elements of communication that are not verbal cover a whole range of behaviours including

- Gesture
- Posture
- Position
- Proximity
- Movement
- Eye contact
- Facial expression

Consider the 'Dos and Don'ts' given in Table 3.1.

Words

The words you speak are clearly important and even when you are using course slides you are in control of what you say. It is never advisable to either read or memorise a script because you are less likely to engage the audience. If you feel the need for security, you

Table 3.1 Dos and Don'ts

	Dos	Don'ts
Gesture	Use natural gestures	Over-exaggerated arm waving
Posture	Look relaxed	Stand rigid; slouch against the wall
Position	Both sides of the room at different times	Hide behind a table or a lectern; stand in the projector beam
Proximity	Close enough	Invade personal space
Movement	Move naturally and purposefully (i.e. to get closer to someone who is asking or answering a question)	Amble aimlessly
Eye contact	Sweep the room at eye level	Gaze at the ceiling or the screen
Facial expression	Look interested; smile	Look bored or irritated
Fixation	Eye contact with the whole room	Get obsessed with someone who answers your first question

might want to put key words on small index cards. In general, however, the slides should be enough to remind you of what you want to say.

Interaction

While the elements described above are extremely important, some attention has to be paid to interaction within your lecture. As we have already discussed, there are serious limitations on what you can achieve by talking alone. However, there may be opportunities within the lecture format to allow an audience to explore and engage with the ideas in conversation with other learners and you as a teacher. Some of these are outlined in Table 3.2.

Questions

Questions are an important way of achieving dialogue and interactivity. They are, however, not quite as simple as they might appear and a bit of background understanding can help the instructor immensely.

Table 3.2 Interactions within the lecture

	Setting the task	Your response
Opportunities to reflect	Think about what I have just told you. How does it fit in with your previous experience? How might you integrate this new approach in your practice?	Taking contributions from enough people to show that you are interested in what they have to say.
Pairs and small group discussion – problem-solving, sharing information or experiences	Talk to your neighbour about the last time you met a similar scenario. What might have improved the outcome?	Recording ideas on flip chart
Prioritising, sequencing, sorting	Look at these features on the screen. What order would you deal with these issues?	Completing a grid on the flipchart – you can be preparing this while they undertake the task

Using questions to determine the level of learning
Bloom et al. (1956) describe six levels in the cognitive domain and there are different ways of asking questions in order to elicit the level you want your audience to engage in as follows:

- *Knowledge*: Seeking factual information, for example '*Where was Sigmund Freud born?*'
- *Comprehension*: Checking understanding, for example '*What contribution did he make to an understanding of the human mind?*'
- *Application*: Exploring the relevance, for example '*How might psychoanalysis impact on the treatment of anxiety and depression among elderly patients?*'
- *Analysis*: Checking the significance, for example '*Talking cures have been superseded to some extent by developments in pharmacology. To what extent to you agree with this statement?*'
- *Synthesis*: Putting knowledge of one subject together with that of another, for example '*In what ways, if any, did the work of Freud change public perception of mental illness.*'
- *Evaluation*: Making comparisons, for example '*Has Freud's contribution to Psychology created a culture in western psychological medicine that is beneficial or trivial?*'

Clearly, some of these questions lend themselves more readily to the seminar rather than the lecture theatre – a further reminder of the limitations of the lecture as a teaching modality.

Methods

Regardless of the level of the question, you can ask them in a number of ways:

Open questions, to the group as a whole: This gives everyone the opportunity to demonstrate their knowledge and insight and if the question has been phrased appropriately and at the right level, there is likely to be someone in the audience who will be able to answer it.

Questions to random, named individuals: This is intended to keep the audience on their toes and attentive to what you are saying. It can, however, be intimidating (and not just to the new learner). Even experienced members of the audience can sometimes be under considerable pressure and may forget things that they would reasonably be expected to know.

Questions along a row: Asking 10 people to name ten known facts has a number of negative effects: the first person has many options open to them, the second person, one less and so on. By the time you get to the eighth person, there are only three left and pressure along the row will almost certainly guarantee that students will not be able to contribute. In the meantime, students in the first few positions can take a break and possibly lose concentration and a sense of engagement.

Pose, pause, pounce: This is a common strategy and it has the merit in encouraging all the audience to think of a possible answer before someone (who may look as if they know) is invited to respond.

Whatever the strategy, there are a number of things you need to do in response to an answer, assuming for the moment that it is correct.

Responses

Acknowledge it: Say 'thank you', rather than 'excellent', 'absolutely' or any other meaningless, over-enthusiastic superlative. A reason for this is that answers to particularly low-level questions are rarely anything other than successfully recalling something from memory – often from another session.

Repeat or paraphrase the answer: some people talk very quietly and other members of the audience may not hear them.

Expand on the response, particularly if it is partial.

Ask supplementary question(s).
Relate it to other parts of your lecture, if relevant.
  Compare:

> *Instructor*: Who can tell me what ABC stands for
> *Student*: Airway, breathing and circulation
> *Instructor*: Excellent!
> *Rest of audience*: (I knew that!)

to:

> *Instructor:* What modifications do you have to make to the Glasgow
>   Coma Score when dealing with a head-injured infant?
> *Audience:* (thinking about it …)
> *Student:* erm, response to voice … can't be the same?
> *Instructor* (nodding and giving eye contact to the respondent): Yes,
>   response to voice. A small infant or baby could not respond
>   articulately to a question. (To the group) Any other thoughts?

Because lectures are rarely introducing new material, and very rarely, complex or abstract material, the likelihood is that respondents will answer correctly. However, you do need to be prepared for two phenomena: the wrong answer and silence. It is important that you allow both, but the strategies are somewhat different. Consider this:

> *Instructor:* Does anyone know the correct dose of amiodarone before
>   the 4th shock in a cardiac arrest?
> *Audience:* (looking at ceiling, fingernails, etc.)
> *Instructor:* Anyone?
> *Student:* 1 mg
> *Instructor:* I think you are probably thinking of adrenaline, but the
>   right answer is 300 mg. It's probably best that you look up doses
>   rather than try to remember them.
> *Audience:* (Phew!)

and

> *Instructor:* OK. Who can tell me what the energy presence, essential for
>   contraction and relaxation of muscle fibres, within cardiac muscles
>   is?

Audience: Silence.

Instructor (after 5 seconds or so): Well, that was a difficult one. The answer is ATP, Adenosine Triphosphate molecules. The way I remember it is that the cardiac muscle fibres are like part of an engine, functional units that still need petrol as the energy source in order for them to work efficiently. ATP is the energy source for cardiac muscles.

Obviously, there should be variations on these, but you should look for the supportive, rather than hypercritical or sarcastic. ('Idiot, you think the first shock should be 50 J? I might need to talk to your clinical director'.) Whatever the strategies you adopt in the dialogue, you should be aiming for a conversation that enables the audience to share with you and everyone else, a more certain understanding of the issues.

Closure

Closure has three stages: asking for questions (and answering them), summarising and termination.

Asking for questions (and waiting for 10 seconds to get any) gives an audience the opportunity to check any uncertainties they may have. In general, it is safe to treat these as genuine requests for information and you answer them briefly and succinctly. You may, however, come across the occasional individual who will ask something like:

Student: I read in a recent edition of the Annals of Emergency Medicine that ...

Invariably, this student is trying to impress you and the rest of the audience, but is unlikely to succeed. However, it is vital that you do not undermine the student (however you might feel) as the question may mask uncertainty and a lack of confidence.

The summary is your opportunity to give the students a 'take-home message' and it should relate directly to the learning outcomes you spelled out in the set. Once more, it should be succinct and not revisit the whole content of what you have had to say. The summary should always follow questions – this ensures that the lecture does not run over time ('I can accept one more question before I summarise') and also ensures that the audience leaves with your take-home message fresh in their mind rather than an awkward question. Termination is important because it avoids the situation in which the audience are not sure what is going to happen next. Something like 'Right, wait here as Professor Angstrom is going to talk to you about a new way of thinking about the control of Type 1 diabetes' or 'Thanks for your attention, and now it's time for coffee. Be back by 11.15'. This is preferable to the audience sitting uncomfortably while the lecturer shuffles papers or recovers a data stick.

Summary and learning

A lecture is an opportunity to remind people of what they may have come across in other contexts and a chance to share issues and concerns within a safe environment. While lectures are not good at delivering complex knowledge or practical skills, they have a distinct place in learning. Using techniques, such as questioning, to engage learners improves the experience.

Reference

Bloom B, Englehart M, Furst E, Hill W, Krathwohl D. *Taxonomy of Educational Objectives: The Classification of Educational Goals. Handbook I: Cognitive Domain.* Longmans, Green, New York, Toronto, 1956.

CHAPTER 4

Teaching skills

Learning outcomes

By the end of this chapter you should be able to demonstrate an understanding of

- the importance of skills teaching
- the four-stage approach to skills teaching
- the use of continuous assessment of skills

Introduction

The development and retention of practical skills is of great importance in many areas of professional life. Once a skill has been learnt, regular practice and improving performance are key factors in developing autonomy. Learners come from varied background and experience, and this is often most apparent by their varied ability to perform the range of key skills.

Acquiring a practical skill is influenced by retention of relevant knowledge, the psychomotor performance and the attitude of the candidate as a learner. The interaction between the candidate and the teaching environment is important in achieving the behavioural change in their practice. The whole process is about promoting independent practice of the skill.

The process of changing behaviour is situation-dependent (in other words, linked to the learners' experiences) as outlined in Chapter 1. The key to success is the instructor's ability to help learners identify how they can apply new information, skills and attitudes to their everyday clinical practice. This familiarity with the context for learning significantly enhances the learning of new skills and greatly increases retention (Ausubel, 1968). Once

Pocket Guide to Teaching for Clinical Instructors, Third Edition.
Edited by Ian Bullock, Mike Davis, Andrew Lockey and Kevin Mackway-Jones.
© 2016 John Wiley & Sons, Ltd. Published 2016 by John Wiley & Sons, Ltd.

this has been established, the skills themselves are best taught in stages. Acquisition of the skill by the candidate reflects their ability to become increasingly organised as a result of the learning experience.

Researchers have demonstrated that retention of both knowledge and psychomotor skills declines sharply after 4–6 months if they are not practised. The retention of skills that are regularly used by clinicians is more encouraging. Thus, over the last decade, we have seen a significant shift from trying to teach all healthcare professionals all domain skills to a more focussed approach on skills that they will use in their normal work. This leads to an increased motivation and desire to learn, with learners realising the value of new skills, which enable them to function in everyday work situations.

Important principles when teaching practical skills are to
- Teach progressively from the simple to the complex
- Teach skills in the order in which they will be used
- Teach one technique at a time
- Employ continual reinforcement
- Follow learning with practice
- Integrate cognitive and psychomotor learning
- Encourage confident employment of the skills

Poor retention of resuscitation skills by learners is attributed in many studies to ineffective teaching. The goal of teaching (or the learning outcome) should change the behaviour of the learner; repeated practice will greatly enhance achievement and performance. The four-stage approach is the teaching methodology adopted on many life support courses and is centred on the way information is processed by the candidate, and not just the factual information provided (Bullock, 2000).

Skills teaching is based on the structured approach. As discussed in Chapter 2, this consists of environment, set, dialogue (where a four-stage approach is used) and closure.

Environment

Preparation of the environment in which the skills are taught is essential if the session is to be successful. Often, several groups are taught in the same room, and therefore, care must be taken to avoid distractions between groups, either by adequate physical separation or by the use of screens. Learners must also have enough room to observe the skill as it is demonstrated. Bodies generate heat and a room containing several groups will soon become hot and stuffy.

As the instructor, it is your responsibility to ensure that you have all the equipment needed to teach the skill. You should ensure that it functions and you know how it works. Arrange the equipment in a realistic manner and remove anything that is not essential.

Set

As explored in Chapter 2, instructors need to introduce themselves and invite students to do the same. They must be given clear, realistic learning outcomes for the session, including the role of continuous assessment in the session. Motivate them by explaining the skill's importance and put it into context within the rest of the course. Finally, be clear about how the learners will be expected to participate in the session. This is vitally important in skills teaching because the approach used may be very different to what they have experienced previously.

Dialogue

This is the part of the session where the skill is actually taught using the four-stage approach. Although all methods of education are ultimately about the processing of information, the four-stage approach is orientated specifically towards developing the learner's ability to acquire and operate on the information received. The four parts are shown in Box 4.1.

Box 4.1 Four-stage technique for skills teaching

Stage 1   Demonstration of the skill, performed at real speed with or without speech.

Stage 2   Repeat demonstration with dialogue, providing the rationale for actions.

Stage 3   Repeat demonstration guided by one or more of the learners.

Stage 4   Repeat demonstration by the learner, and practice of the skill by all learners.

The skills teaching algorithm
Stage 1

Animating clinical expertise. Demonstration of the skill, performed at real speed with or without speech.

In this first stage, the instructor demonstrates the skill as they would normally practise it. In order to create realism, the demonstration is performed in real time, allowing the learner a unique 'fly-on-the-wall' view of the performance of the skill. No commentary or explanation is given, but any verbalisation that accompanies the skill, for example shouting for help during basic life support, should be included. The demonstration provides the candidate with strong visual imagery which shapes new learning.

Stage 2

> Reinforcing components of clinical expertise. Repeat demonstration with dialogue, providing the rationale for actions.

During this stage, there is an exchange of facts and ideas between teacher and learners. In stage 2, the instructor slows down the performance of the skill and provides a description of actions and indicates briefly, where necessary, the evidence base for the skill where appropriate: in other words, the 'what' and 'why'. Involving the candidate and acknowledging what they bring to the learning environment increases their motivation and desire to learn. This allows the instructor to lead them from what they already know to what they need to know. A period of time for questions within stage 2 is important to enable the learners to gain clarity and the instructor to assess understanding prior to stage 3.

Stage 3

> Part transition of responsibility for the skill from instructor to candidate. Repeat demonstration guided by one of the learners.

During this third stage, a learner (or learners) talks the instructor through the skill while the instructor performs it. This allows learners to 'Gather and organise information from the environment in order to form useful patterns, which form the basis of their own future behaviour' (Eggen and Kauchek, 1998). Strong visual reminders will help the candidate recall the skill under the stressful conditions of actual practice.

At this stage the responsibility for the performed skill is moved gently away from the instructor towards the learner. The emphasis here is on cognitive understanding (knowledge) that will guide the psychomotor activity (performance of the skill) in stage 4. The instructor must ensure that the candidate is supported as he/she takes the lead in talking the instructor through the skills; it may be necessary to give the student doing the talk through visual or verbal clues as to the next appropriate step. It is also important at stage 3 (and indeed at stage 4) to correct any errors or misapprehensions. Opportunity for further questions and reflection on the skill adds to this stage. Positive reinforcement of good practice will enhance the future practice of each individual learner.

Stage 4

Independent candidate practice. Repeat demonstration by the learner and practise of the skill by all learners.

This stage completes the teaching and learning process and allows each learner to practise the particular skill. For virtually all newly learned skills, a single practice will be insufficient, and all learners must be encouraged to continue to practise in order to gain further confidence and competence until eventually mastery is achieved. Once learners have demonstrated competence in a particular skill they should be encouraged to maintain this level of performance throughout the rest of the course, reinforcing skilled practice.

Closure

Although most of the questions generated during the skills teaching session will have been raised and answered during stages 3 and 4, it is essential that an opportunity be given for final questions to be aired. A summary should affirm achievement of the objectives for the session, linking the skill to the rest of the course and reinforcing its importance and usefulness.

Summary and learning

This well-structured and systematic approach allows repeat practice of skills in a safe environment.

The four-stage approach to skills teaching is promoted. The main focus of using this methodology is to transfer skill from the expert (instructor) to the novice (candidate), as steps towards achieving competence.

References

Ausubel D. *Educational Psychology: A Cognitive View.* Holt, Rinehart and Winston, New York, 1968.

Bullock I. Skill acquisition in resuscitation. *Resuscitation,* 2000;45:139–143.

Eggen PD, Kauchek DP. *Strategies for Teachers. Teaching Content and Thinking Skills.* Prentice Hall, Englewood Cliffs, NJ, 1998.

CHAPTER 5

Managing simulations

Learning outcomes

By the end of this chapter you should be able to demonstrate an understanding of
- the purpose of simulation
- the origins of simulation
- the management of simulation

Introduction

Simulation teaching is based on the notion of 'let's pretend … ' or more seriously 'a willing suspension of disbelief' within which learners step outside of their own experiences and try out behaviours, perhaps at the edge of their comfort zone. To achieve this, they have to play roles.

There are five common types of role-play:

- *Improvisation*: Learners use their own responses and actions in a given situation; in other words, they behave as themselves but in a novel (to them) context. For example 'You are in the bar at the theatre when an old man nearby clutches his chest and falls to the floor … '.
- *Structured*: Learners are given a role to play with clear instructions on how this should be performed. For example 'You are a nervous junior doctor confronted with a febrile child and her mother … '.
- *Prepared improvisation*: As with improvisation but following a discussion as to the nature of the roles, and possible outcomes.

Pocket Guide to Teaching for Clinical Instructors, Third Edition.
Edited by Ian Bullock, Mike Davis, Andrew Lockey and Kevin Mackway-Jones.
© 2016 John Wiley & Sons, Ltd. Published 2016 by John Wiley & Sons, Ltd.

- *Reverse role-play*: When learners play a role other than their normal one to gain insight into the thoughts, attitudes and behaviours of others, for example the learner might play the role of a parent being informed about a serious illness in their baby.
- *Exaggerated role-play*: Over-developing the features of a character to make a particular point, for example, an aggressive relative receiving bad news.

Role-play can also be used to teach specific interpersonal skills, which may then later be included in more complex simulations. For example, telephone discussions with a senior clinician about a referral may be conducted by seating two learners back-to-back.

As with all teaching modalities, attention has to be paid to planning and facilitation, with attention to environment and set being central to the success of the subsequent dialogue. There are differences between the two, largely arising from the fact that role-plays tend to be free of equipment while simulations rely on a more complex environment.

Simulations (sometimes called moulages and previously called scenarios) are focused role-play sessions often used in healthcare teaching.

Jones (1987) defines a simulation as

> ... *an untaught event in which sufficient information is provided to allow the participants to achieve reality of function in a simulated environment.*

Presented in these terms, simulation teaching can overcome some of the traditional reservations about this form of teaching by emphasising emotional security (see Maslow in Chapter 1).

More importantly, simulations have the capacity to recognise and build on the learning that takes place in the work-setting: the ward, the emergency department or the pre-hospital environment. This acknowledges the understanding we have of learning arising from situated cognition, a theory of learning which was explored in Chapter 1.

Simulations have the capacity to allow learners to integrate their learning from other contexts: reading, lectures, skills stations and workshops. In something approaching real time, learners can interact within a context, including other health professionals and relevant equipment (ECG, tubes, collars, etc.); with manikins or actors; and with instructors who provide clinical and other information and prompt learners as to the correct way in which to assess a patient and to make decisions in a way that is, as far as possible, true to life.

At the heart of simulation teaching is role-play in which learners act out how to behave in a clinical case. In the case of learners on life support courses, the expectation is that the role they play is that of themselves. In other words, they improvise actions but based on their usual behaviour in a novel context.

Environment

The complexity of the environment will depend on the nature of the simulation. Attention has to be paid, therefore, to creating an environment that will allow learners to demonstrate their skills, knowledge and affect. Accordingly, fixtures and fittings, furniture and clinical equipment will have to be both present and tested. You might also need to consider:

- *Privacy*: Being overlooked by people external to the immediate group.
- *Proximity*: How close do you want people to be to one another?
- *Eye lines*: Do you want observers to be in direct eye line with the main participants? Simulation suites now allow audience viewing either through one-way mirrors or via high-quality audio-visual links to minimise this issue.

Even though simulation is not *real*, it does need to be *realistic* and this also needs careful planning. Much of that, however, will be built into the design of the event and that is beyond the scope of this chapter. Where you can ensure some fidelity, however, is by ensuring that individuals are given roles they could reasonably be expected to play, within a context that they have some familiarity: a junior trainee in Emergency Medicine might struggle to role-play a consultant paediatrician discussing possible child abuse with parents. The role description and the context should be enough to enable the role-players to explore the issues experientially within a constrained period of time followed by shared reflection about what took place.

It is vital that the simulation is properly explored in order for everyone (active participants and observers) to learn from it. Time management is something that you need to emphasise, so that the learners know how long they have got and that you will let them know when they need to move towards closure.

Set

The instructor needs to be particularly clear about the roles of participants, the degree of simulation fidelity and the learning outcomes for the session. As discussed below it is very important that the way in which information is to be shared during the simulation is understood by all those participating and this should be clearly stated.

Dialogue

As you will recognise from earlier chapters, the dialogue is the main component of the teaching episode, and in the case of simulation, this involves the candidates engaging actively with the management of a clinical case.

As is explored in the introduction to this chapter, this involves a degree of make-believe and there are two elements that contribute towards this:

- structural fidelity
- functional fidelity

Structural fidelity is realised in the way in which equipment is provided. This can be low, medium or high fidelity, depending on the resources that are available to a centre. In most cases of life support training, equipment is likely to be medium fidelity: manikins will have some capacity to replicate the human body as airway, breathing and circulation are managed. This may be supplemented by monitors of various levels of fidelity. As far as possible, all appropriate equipment should be available to allow the candidates to manage the case.

To some extent, however, structural fidelity is not as important as functional fidelity and it has been argued that high fidelity equipment can be a distraction (Norman et al., 2012).

Functional fidelity or more helpfully "psychological realism" is a more important ingredient in that a high level of physical realism is not always essential to deliver a good educational outcome. For example, human factors training can be successfully achieved with low fidelity manikins.

Nevertheless, it is worth exploring each type of realism in turn.

Physical realism

There can be different levels of fidelity depending on the availability of manikins:

- High fidelity – computer-controlled simulator with the capability to simulate: voice, heart sounds, breath sounds, chest rise, palpable pulses, cardiovascular monitoring with vital signs, fluid administration and fluid loss.

- Low or medium fidelity – any other simulator that does not meet all of the requirements of a high fidelity simulator. For many years, low-to-medium fidelity simulators have been used for simulation teaching. They have the advantage that they are cheap and readily available. They are ideal for teaching situations where a patient is not expected to have any vital signs (e.g. basic life support for cardiac arrest). In these simulations, the instructor is required to verbally supply any information about the patient to the candidate. Failure to do this in a timely manner can reduce the psychological realism.

Medium-to-high fidelity manikins are now available that enable candidates to measure physiological variables directly and also interact verbally with the manikin. Some of these manikins can be controlled wirelessly, enabling them to be placed in real-life clinical environments. This added fidelity enables simulations to highlight actual problems that need rectifying.

The main disadvantages with medium-to-high fidelity manikins are their cost and the potential for malfunction. There is no convincing evidence that the use of these manikins for teaching on life support courses improves patient outcomes or indeed candidate performance, although it may be a more enjoyable teaching modality for students.

The use of live patients (actors or real patients) is the ultimate in high fidelity simulation and can provide some considerable advantages, but also some disadvantages. These are summarised in Box 5.1.

Box 5.1 Comparison of manikins and real patient or actors

	Low fidelity manikin	Medium fidelity manikin	Real patient or actor
Realism			✓ ✓
Appearance	✓	✓	✓ ✓
Verbal/physical interaction			✓ ✓
Procedure performance	✓ ✓	✓ ✓	
Safety	✓ ✓	✓ ✓	✓

Among the difficulties presented by real patients or actors is the need to behave realistically. Thus they need to be carefully briefed and must practise the simulation so that difficulties can be resolved. If they are made up so that they look as if they have the illness or trauma that they are supposed to have, this may add to the learner's experience. Of course it is not always possible to practise invasive skills on live patients.

Psychological realism

Much of the psychological realism is premised on the fact that the clinical case that is being simulated is something that candidates might encounter in their working lives. As such, it has real significance for them and their practice,

In a rapid response to a column in the BMJ in 2014, Davis wrote

My observation is that the narrower the experiential gap between learning and application, the more likely there will be higher level transfer. This is supported by two features: effective facilitation of the training event which aims for high levels of psychological realism; and secondly, well designed and effective feedback sessions which encourage self awareness and reflection, which the authors recognise as being essential ingredients of good practice. The curriculum, therefore, is not content based but dependent on an authentic process designed to encourage self-knowledge.

It is important that clinical information flow is delivered in real time. If the simulation is utilising a low fidelity manikin, the responsibility for providing this appropriately belongs to the instructor running the scenario. It is better to be proactive, rather than reactive, thus

---

Learner (to helper): Could you check blood pressure?
(pause)
Learner (to instructor): What's the blood pressure?
Instructor: 90 over 70.

---

as opposed to:

Learner (to helper): Could you check blood pressure?
(pause)
Instructor: 90 over 70.

In the second example, the instructor is providing clinical information in real time, thereby adding to the psychological reality of the simulation. The role of the instructor in a simulation is to provide this clinical information and offer the occasional prompt in order to help the learner keep within the protocols. These should be subtle, for example:

'What do you think should happen next?'

as opposed to:

'Do you think you should move onto circulation now?'

There are a number of issues in the way in which the instructor can help manage the candidate's experience and these are intended to allow the exercise of imagination to 'fill in the gaps' of the physical reality. Two non-clinical references may help clarify what is meant here. The first is from Kurt Lewin, writing in 1951 about how groups function. He writes:

> *Our behavior is purposeful; we live in a psychological reality or life space that includes not only those parts of our physical and social environment that are important to us but also imagined states that do not currently exist.*
> *Kurt Lewin (1951)*

The playwright Brian Friel represents this view in a similar way:

> *... what fascinates me about that memory is that it owes nothing to fact. In that memory, atmosphere is more real than incident and everything is simultaneously actual and illusory. Dancing at Lughnasa, Brian Friel (1988)*

The capacity of candidates to engage fully with an effectively managed, low fidelity simulation is widely experienced on life support courses, and the instructor's role is intended to help them make effective use of this engagement.

As part of this, the instructor has the responsibility to manage time flow. Some learners may be slow and they need to be prompted by adding in new, and possibly urgent, clinical signs (e.g. 'the patient is losing consciousness'). Others may move rapidly, usually by telling the instructor what they would do, rather than actually doing it. The latter can be controlled by simple requests, for example:

> *Learner*: I would get in two lines, measure cap refill and get blood pressure.
> *Instructor*: Show me.

Remember, the simulation is an integration of skills and knowledge acquired elsewhere and learners should be encouraged to demonstrate their psychomotor ability as well as their knowledge.

During the simulation itself, the instructor is there to provide clinical signs where necessary, to prompt, if required, to listen and to manage time boundaries. It might be helpful to make notes to assist the discussion that follows, which is also part of the dialogue. This is explored in more detail in Chapter 8.

A note on safety

Among the concerns associated with simulation teaching is that of safety, particularly in the context of defibrillation or the safe use/disposal of sharps. Sessions should be terminated immediately in the event of safety being compromised.

Closure

As discussed earlier in this chapter, simulation teaching has a strong emotional component and participants need to be allowed to return to normal, particularly if they have been dealing with issues that could resonate powerfully with their own experience.

As with all teaching modalities, simulations need to close properly, by:

- Inviting questions or comments about the issues that have emerged.
- Offering a summary of the learning that has taken place – often by revisiting the learning outcomes offered in the set.
- Terminating the session and moving learners on to the next event.

Summary and learning

Simulation teaching differs from other teaching methods in the way in which, if successful, it relates directly to practice. It utilises skills, knowledge and affect in order to enable learners to explore a simulation of their real world.

As an instructor, you should aspire to make the simulations as psychologically real as necessary to maximise the learning experience for all participants.

References

Bullock I, Davis M, Lockey A, Mackway-Jones K. *Pocket Guide to Teaching for Medical Instructors*. Blackwell, Oxford, 2008.

Davis MP, Navathe AS, Janin SH. Medical education's authenticity problem. *BMJ*, 2014;348:g2651.

Friel B. *Dancing at Lughnasa*. Faber and Faber, London, 1990.

Hamstra SJ, Brydges R, Hatala R, Zendejas B, Cook DA. Reconsidering fidelity in simulation-based training. *Academic Medicine*, 2014;89(3):1–6.

Jones K. *Simulations: A Handbook for Teachers and Trainers*, 2nd ed. Kogan Page, London, 1987.

Lewin K. *Field Theory in Social Science: Selected Theoretical Papers*. In: Cartwright D, ed. Harper & Row, New York, 1951.

Norman G, Dore K, Grierson L. The minimal relationship between simulation fidelity and transfer of learning. *Medical Education*, 2012;46:636–647.

CHAPTER 6
Facilitating discussions

Learning outcomes

By the end of this chapter you should be able to demonstrate an understanding of
- group dynamics
- the different ways of facilitating group discussions
- open and closed facilitation

Introduction

Working in groups can be an extremely effective method of learning, particularly for professionals in a multidisciplinary environment. The outcomes of well-organised group activity can be better than those achieved by an individual member working alone. It is also recognised that group activity can be extremely useful in assessing adults' ability to apply theoretical knowledge to practice. To achieve these goals this teaching method requires the teacher to be a facilitator of learning rather than a definitive source of knowledge. The challenge therefore is to create a setting where learners benefit from a more student-centred experience than, say, a lecture, however interactive that might be.

As explored in Chapter 1, adults bring a wealth of personal experience to the classroom and it is important to recognise and build on this; group activities allow this far better than many other approaches. As with all educational activities, good planning, organisation and facilitation are required. The ideal group size is between four and twelve for discussions. If the group is too small, discussion can be difficult to start. Participants can become

Pocket Guide to Teaching for Clinical Instructors, Third Edition.
Edited by Ian Bullock, Mike Davis, Andrew Lockey and Kevin Mackway-Jones.
© 2016 John Wiley & Sons, Ltd. Published 2016 by John Wiley & Sons, Ltd.

inactive and contribute less if the group is larger and there is greater potential for sub-group formation.

This chapter explores the different approaches to group discussions, providing some ideas for their planning while highlighting the skills required in facilitating them. Though the skills used in running discussions are those of a facilitator, the term 'instructor' will be used throughout, encompassing the roles of teacher and facilitator.

Effective planning is crucial. The first stage is to clearly define the desired outcomes of the session, as this will determine which type of group session you will run. Historically, we talked about 'open' and 'closed' discussions, but we are now not making this distinction. There is, however, recognition that some subjects lend themselves to more open-ended outcomes than others, for example compare two discussions: 'Elicitation of 4Hs and 4Ts during cardiac arrest' and 'An exploration of the presence of relatives during a child's resuscitation'.

In the former there is a right answer, while in the latter, there are good answers, but there are other answers that have merit.

As with all of the teaching modalities, attention needs to be paid to four elements:

- Environment
- Set
- Dialogue
- Closure

Environment

Apart from the usual considerations of heat, light, comfort and so on, the environment is primarily concerned with seating layout and where any relevant audio-visual aid is positioned. Common aids used to focus the discussion are flip charts, laptops, whiteboards or overhead projectors. Increasingly, some instructors are making use of tablets and designated software suitable for sharing images and other slide content.

Figure 6.1 shows a possible layout for seating in a discussion that enables all candidates to see and contribute.

Set

In some respects, the set is the most important contribution that the instructor makes in small group discussions. Some of this is obvious (i.e. outlining the intended learning outcomes); others are quite subtle, demanding as much attention to paralinguistic

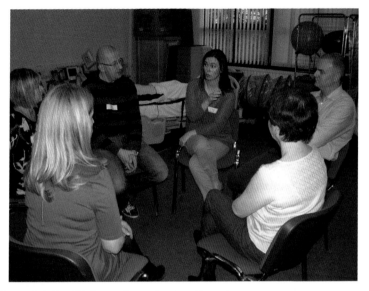

Figure 6.1 Possible layout for seating in a discussion

behaviour as what is said. It is helpful to include quick introductions, which serve two purposes:
- It gives everyone the opportunity to 'hear their voice' in the group. This allows them to claim 'air time' and gives them permission to speak again
- It allows the facilitator to make some assessment of the group's individual and collective experience and affect.

In creating a purposeful mood, the instructor puts some effort into moving quickly and succinctly to the subject under consideration. Quite considerable thought needs to go into the opening comments and questions and in planning the nature of the questions you pose; you need to have in mind the cognitive hierarchy, explored in Chapter 1. It is worth revisiting this here:

Cognitive needs (to know and understand)
Different levels of cognition: • Knowledge • Comprehension • Application • Analysis • Synthesis • Evaluation

It will be clear to you that if your opening question is a knowledge-level question, there is not going to be much discussion. For example '*What is the capital of Norway?*'

Equally, if you ask a very high-level question (synthesis of evaluation), it may be beyond all or most of your group. For example '*What is the meaning of life?*'

Often, then, questions pitched at the level of

Comprehension
• 'What do you understand by … ',

Application
• 'Has anyone had any experience of … '
• 'What do others think? ' or

Analysis
• 'Now we have explored this case, what are the implications of accurate diagnosis?'

are what is required to encourage the candidates to engage with one another. The most important feature of a discussion is that it is an opportunity for the group to talk to one another, rather than listen to the facilitator, which is why the nature of the questions you ask is so important. David Kolb, an American social scientist famous for introducing the 'experiential learning cycle' (see Chapter 1) talked at a conference in Finland about the nature of facilitation and related it to the notion of the dinner party host. In Kolb's view, this role was to create an environment, provide food and drink and invite the right combination of guests. The role during dinner was more enabling: ensuring food and drink arrived in a timely manner, gently refereeing, when required, and bringing the evening to a satisfactory conclusion.

Dialogue

This metaphor may help you think through the process of small group management. The key element to keep in mind is that you should not be the centre of attention; rather you should be a relatively silent presence, who listens attentively and contributes when necessary, in order to redirect, refocus or bring to a conclusion. The most common pitfall for the instructor in discussions is the temptation to deliver a lecture to a small group. If, at the end of your session, you realise that you have talked more than 10% of the time, your session might have been more about you as a facilitator than it is about participants as learners.

Group dynamics and candidate behaviour
Managing discussions can be quite complex. The instructor's role is to pose the problem and allow students to explore their understanding. An effective discussion requires group members to have done some preparation by pre-reading and the purpose of the discussion is to check their understanding and clarify any uncertainties through discussion among themselves. As we have explored above, the role of the instructor is more of a participant – observer during these sessions. After the initial questions, a subtle use of body language and a particular approach to asking questions (see below), allow the conversation to develop among the candidates, having them speaking to one another, rather than directing everything to you. This saves you from occupying a judicial role, which is something that can be observed in adult education settings where sessions become

> ... *emotional battlegrounds with members vying for recognition and affirmation from each other and from the discussion leader.* (Brookfield, 1993)

This is the socio-emotional component of the learning environment and, unless it is well handled, can interfere with effective learning for many group members. More significantly, however, it is the nature of the interactions that is expected among the group. The question we should consider is
• What is the nature of the intellectual activity that candidates are engaging in?
In lectures, this is relatively straightforward: candidates listen, consider, compare with existing knowledge and either accept or reject the conclusions – usually the former. In discussion, however, it is not simply a matter of rehearsing what has been previously read. As Candy puts it:

> *If cognitive process are indeed processes of reconstruction rather than replicating or depicting an a priori existing reality, then the focus of any explanatory effort must shift from what there is or may be to how we arrive at the conceptual constructs we actually have.* (Candy, 1991)

Paralinguistic behaviour
As explored in Chapter 3, some experts in communication argue that body language communicates more than words. Certainly some unconscious behaviours can communicate very effectively

and particular attention needs to be paid to these to avoid negative impact on the group. Some helpful strategies include

- Make frequent sweeps of the group at eye level but do not give eye contact to a person who is speaking. This might sound hostile or aggressive, but it makes people speak to the group rather than to you.
- Sit back after your initial statement and subsequent questions.
- Be aware of encouraging learners to believe that you validate contributions by nodding or saying 'excellent' or similar – doing this may encourage the group to believe they have found the right answer and the discussion will have come to an end without all candidates having had time to contribute and to think it through.

Potential issues

The issue that is of most concern to facilitators of interactive sessions is that of control: that if the group is encouraged to talk amongst themselves, instructors will lose control and chaos will reign. This is usually down to expectations/fears about certain candidate types and these have been summarised as talkers, non-talkers and destroyers (Mackway-Jones and Walker, 1999). Destroyers are extremely rare, the other two more common.

You want people to talk. If, however, some people talk too much, you can impact on their behaviour by

- not giving eye contact (see above)
- turning away slightly so you are orientated towards another part of the group
- raising a hand (palm up) – see Figure 6.2
- asking 'What do other people think?'
- saying 'Hang on a second, [name]'

It takes a determined talker to continue over the top of those cues.

On the other hand, non-talkers can be encouraged by

- giving eye contact
- turning towards that person
- offering an open hand – see Figure 6.3
- asking 'Does anyone on this side of the room have any experience?'
- saying '[name], as an ED registrar, you must have come across similar cases'

It is not essential, however, for everyone to make a contribution as long as they are being attentive.

Small groups lay bare some of the complex socio-psychological issues of teaching and learning, mainly arising from instructors'

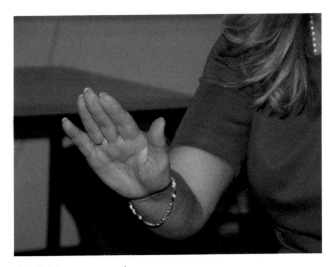

Figure 6.2 Raising an open palm

concerns about power and authority. However, much of the research suggests that among fairly well-motivated communities, group cohesion and a sense of responsibility almost guarantee an emotionally safe environment based on an acceptance that the instructor is the site of power in the group: group members subscribe to this because of their psychological need for safety.

Closure

In this instance, it may not be appropriate to ask if anyone has any questions, but the instructor should ensure that the session is satisfactorily terminated. If the discussion was particularly heated

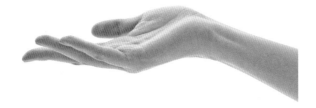

Figure 6.3 Offering an open palm
Source: © ba1ran via iStock/Getty Images.

or if there appear to be some unresolved issues, these should be acknowledged and should be dealt with before terminating the session. Final remarks should include a statement of the progress that has been made

Summary and learning

Well-managed discussions are essentially learner-orientated activities in which the instructor adopts the role of facilitator/host by creating the right environment, posing the right questions and then exercising vigilance, only engaging in speaking when the discussion needs some (re)direction. The effective facilitator trusts the process and the learners soon follow suit.

References

Brookfield S. Through the lens of learning: how the visceral experience of learning reframes teaching. In: Boud D, Cohen R, Walker D, eds. *Using Experience for Learning*. SHRE/Open University, Buckingham, 1993: 24.

Candy P. *Self-direction for Lifelong Learning*. Jossey-Bass, San Francisco, 1991: 273.

Mackway-Jones K, Walker M. *Pocket Guide to Teaching for Medical Instructors*. BMJ Books, London, 1999.

CHAPTER 7

Getting assessment right

Learning outcomes

By the end of this chapter you should be able to demonstrate an understanding of
- what is meant by assessment and its purpose
- different assessment approaches
- how assessment may facilitate learning and predict candidate performance

Introduction

Assessment is one of the most challenging aspects of the education process. It typically provokes high emotional responses from both teachers and learners. It is essential that instructors have a basic understanding of assessment methodology and a good understanding of the particular assessment approaches used on courses, so that assessment tools are properly used. This will help increase the reliability of assessments actually reflecting the learner's ability (Perkins, 2001). The purpose of this chapter is to define the educational principles that lie behind the assessment techniques used.

What do we mean by assessment?

In education, the term assessment is used to describe the process of evaluating or making a judgement about a student's ability. This process involves collecting data, observing and measuring

Pocket Guide to Teaching for Clinical Instructors, Third Edition.
Edited by Ian Bullock, Mike Davis, Andrew Lockey and Kevin Mackway-Jones.
© 2016 John Wiley & Sons, Ltd. Published 2016 by John Wiley & Sons, Ltd.

performance and interpreting information about the outcome of an educational process. This can be focused on an individual or on a group of candidates.

Methods of assessment used are based on principles well defined in educational practice and involve the evaluation of the candidate's performance against pre-set criteria. Both written and practical assessments of knowledge and skills can be undertaken; in all cases the assessor is required to make a judgement about the candidate's performance. The outcome will be more consistent and reproducible when the answer is clear-cut as in a multiple choice question (MCQ) paper. The cognitive domain is often tested through the MCQ, which delivers a summative judgement on a learner's ability to recall knowledge. In practical skills or simulated settings, the assessment depends more on subjective opinion that the assessor makes about the candidate's performance against some pre-set criteria. Assessors need to understand very clearly their own responsibilities in the process as well as the issues that the candidates themselves face. The qualities of an expert assessor have been described by Laryea (1994):

> You need a sense of fairness and willingness to treat people as candidates and not entities. You should not behave in a manner that may create anxiety in the individual that you are assessing. You are not there to fail a person, but to help them realise their potential.

Given this description, the challenge is to ensure that any assessment process actually measures what it is supposed to. In other words, within the context of a training course, it is fit for the purpose of indicating how the candidate will react in a real situation.

Summative assessment (e.g. MCQ)
Assessment using a single testing approach of learning that has taken place and counts towards an overall mark at the end of the period of study.

Continuous assessment (e.g. skills)
An ongoing process throughout the duration of the course, involving repeated sampling of a candidate's practice, providing more realistic assessment. Skills are initially assessed using outcome-based methods and then repeatedly observed throughout the course.

Why assess?

The reasons why we assess are
- to quantify or measure candidate achievement
- to support learning as an iterative process (particularly within the context of blended learning)
- to focus and motivate the candidate
- to measure the effectiveness of teaching and learning
- to provide evidence to inform feedback for the student and teacher
- to predict candidate performance when in work-based situations.

Assessment traditionally has been viewed as something that happens after learning has taken place. However, assessment is integral to a candidate's learning (Jarvis, 1995). It can start in a VLE, providing iterative feedback that affirms, shapes and corrects learner understanding. It continues in lecture-based presentations and is applied in individual skill and non-technical skill situations, leading to confidence in practice and an appreciation of the clinical situation.

Assessment design

Getting assessment right is a key aim for instructors, and performance here is as important as delivering a good lecture, providing iterative feedback in a virtual environment, facilitating a workshop or creating a simulated clinical environment. Candidates should feel confident that decisions reached during assessments are consistent and fair. The following have been identified as particularly important in achieving this goal.

Validity, which is concerned with the content of the examination:
- Are the right things being assessed?
- Is the assessment a fair test?
- Does success in the assessment predict good future performance?

Reliability, which is concerned with the accuracy of the assessment:
- Is the assessment passing and failing the right candidates?
- Do different instructors agree with each other?
- Would the candidate obtain a similar result if re-tested without additional learning?

Feasibility, which is the balance between reliability and validity, measured against practical assessment issues (time and resources available).

Specificity, which relates to the method of assessment chosen:
• The assessment should be relevant to the skill or area of learning being assessed.

Fidelity, which is the closeness to reality (physical and/or functional) of the assessment experience:
• The assessment must be as realistic as possible.

Assessment can also conform to the 'Environment, Set, Dialogue, Closure' approach, even when continuous assessment is the overarching assessment methodology.

Environment

For an assessment to maximise its effectiveness, the environment should be one that is conducive to achieving the points in the previous section. Therefore, an area that allows quiet and uninterrupted performance will afford the learners the optimum environment for assessment. For an MCQ this is easily achieved by allocating a quiet room with adequate seating where candidates have room to spread out without fear of being overlooked by other candidates. Placing signs outside stating 'Quiet Please Exam in Progress' may also help reduce the extraneous noise that is often present in a hospital or educational setting. Ensuring a clock is visible and that there are pens/pencils and enough examination question and answer papers to hand are also key parts of paper-based assessment. For other methods of assessment, it is still important to create an environment that promotes a professional approach. Some centres have flimsy dividing curtain between teaching/assessing stations and the resultant noise pollution can be extremely distracting for candidates and faculty alike. Best practice is to have dedicated rooms for each skill station or simulation so that assessments can be carried out without excess noise, interruption or distraction.

Another important element of assessment is making sure that all equipment is working and programmed correctly for the skill or simulation. Equipment malfunction or instructor error in assessment may severely affect a candidate's performance and invalidate that assessment necessitating a repeat performance, which serves to increase anxiety and should be avoided where possible.

Set

The key element in set is stating that an assessment is being conducted. For the MCQ or simulation test, this may seem fairly obvious, but it still needs to be stated that this is an assessment. This is often done by the Course Director during the introductory session, but candidates should be aware when assessment decisions are being made about them. They should also know the criteria upon which they are being assessed so that the standard expected of them is explicit. For formal examinations such as MCQ, this is simply the pass mark required and time frame to complete the examination. For skills and simulations, it would often be inappropriate and/or impractical to show the candidates the assessment criteria, but they should be aware what you are assessing, e.g. airway management, communication skills, initial assessment and cardiac arrest management.

Set also involves setting the mood without intimidating candidates and making sure that fellow instructors or helpers are clearly briefed on the assessment process and their roles therein. Mentors can help prepare learners for assessment situations by explaining processes and discussing insecurities.

Finally, set should include a description of what will happen during the assessment so that the candidates are absolutely clear about the process they are about to experience. For some assessment situations, this will include telling them that they will be asked to leave the room while the assessors confer about the outcome.

Dialogue

The dialogue is the assessment performance by the candidate. For MCQ, it starts when you say 'turn your papers over' at which point it is up to the individual candidate to answer the questions to the best of their ability. Of course there should always be an invigilator present to answer any practical questions that the candidates may have (not to help answer the questions). A supportive, not directive, role is therefore required. This is similar for the other forms of assessment. In skills or communication stations the instructor must guide the dialogue without being directive in order to allow candidates to achieve the assessment outcomes without direct prompting. This provides evidence of independent practice and helps achieve a more valid assessment.

Dialogue may include asking the candidate questions to clarify intent. For example, 'What are you thinking now?' is appropriate, whereas 'Is there anything else you want to do now?' implies they have missed something and may be directing or pointing them to a particular treatment strategy. As stated above, all those involved in assessment should know their role and give appropriate feedback to candidates if questioned. Candidate – 'Is that tube in the right place?' Instructor/Helper – 'I saw it go through the cords' should still prompt the candidate to verify correct placement, whereas 'It's in!' would make the candidate assume that the manikin has been intubated correctly. This may be fine if airway management is not key to progression of the simulation, but if airway problems need to be specifically identified as key treatment points, it may deflect the candidate from reaching those key points as they may assume all is being satisfactorily dealt with.

These subtleties of assessment take time to master and therefore the inexperienced instructor should be reticent in conducting assessments, especially with candidates who are known to be struggling. Try to avoid superlatives or affirmative words or phrases – 'Brilliant!' 'Well done!' 'Good' 'That was fabulous, just take a step outside while we discuss your performance'. Obviously, if these phrases are delivered and the candidate then fails to achieve the assessment outcomes, it sends a rather confusing message to the candidate.

Closure

In assessment, closure starts with termination and ends with results. The earlier one can give results, the better. We have already discussed how adults need timely feedback and for an assessment this, for the candidate, is whether they have passed or not. For examinations, this follows marking; for simulation testing, it occurs after conferring with co-instructors; and for other elements, it may occur after faculty meetings or discussions. Mentors and/or assessors must relay relevant information on performance to candidates as soon as practicably possible. The assessors do not enter into a learning conversation with candidates after assessment, they merely state 'Well done you passed' or 'I'm afraid you did not pass that test for the following reasons ... '. Opportunities for re-tests, repeating elements of the course and extra supervised practice differ from course to course and should always be clarified with the Course Director before you embark on assessments.

In assessment stations where the whole group is involved, some subtlety in managing the failing candidate is required. The candidates who achieved the assessment outcomes must be told in a timely manner, as should those that failed to meet those criteria. For these latter candidates, a 'tap on the shoulder' at the end of a session allows you to draw them away from the rest of the group in order discuss their performance in privacy and give timely feedback on their level of attainment.

The easiest course closures are those where all candidates have passed and the Course Director can say, at the end and before individual results are handed out by mentors, 'Well, done you have all passed!' Of course this does not always happen and individual results must be delivered to all candidates so that they are clear of their position before they leave the venue. Argumentative or disgruntled candidates are best directed to the Course Director so that any issues can be resolved while the faculty is still present.

Failure to pass a course does not necessarily mean that the candidate has failed to learn. Many candidates with the right support and approach will benefit and learn a great deal, and their practice may improve in consequence. Assessment is not and should not be made a measure of a candidate's worth in their occupational role; it is merely a reflection of their ability to demonstrate specific learning outcomes in a particular way at a particular time. Being able to do this is as much about the ability of the instructor to teach as it is of the candidate to learn.

Summary and learning

The assessment of candidates is a fundamental part of an instructor's role. Its purpose is to facilitate the process of learning and to ensure that high standards are maintained. This may start in a VLE through iterative feedback, laying a foundation for face-to-face teaching and learning.

Assessment should be carefully planned to reflect the content and teaching approach within the curriculum. Getting assessment right facilitates both the candidates' personal and professional development. Enabling instructors to understand and develop confidence in assessment is an important element in measuring the quality of the candidate experience and the course undertaken.

References

Jarvis P. *Adult and Continuing Education: Theory and Practice.* Routledge, London, 1995.

Laryea P. In: Parsloe E, ed. *Coaching, Mentoring and Assessing: A Practical Guide to Developing Competence.* Kogan Page, London, 1994.

Perkins GD, Hulme J, Tweed MJ. Variability in the assessment of advanced life support skills. *Resuscitation* 2001;50(3):281–286.

CHAPTER 8
Feedback

Learning outcomes

By the end of this chapter you will be able to demonstrate an understanding of
- feedback and its contribution to learning

Introduction

Feedback has increasingly become the focus of good educational practice because of the opportunity it provides for learners to reflect and at the same time receive quality input into aspects of their performance. Its purpose is to help learners achieve autonomy in the target field, acquiring along the way appropriate cognitive, psychomotor and affective characteristics. In order to be effective the process needs to be sensitive, relevant and useful: the challenge is to find the appropriate language to enable this to happen.

Feedback has gone through a number of phases in recent years, emphasising results, self-esteem or dialogue. An example of feedback focussed on self-esteem and praise is based on ideas suggested by Pendleton et al. (1984) as illustrated in Figure 8.1. An example of a dialogic approach is the learning conversation (see Figure 8.2).

There are significant advantages from using an approach based on dialogue with the learner. Saunders and Gowing (1999) found that students favoured 'a mutual discussion of the work rather than [being] exposed to one-sided evaluation and criticism', while Juwah et al. (2004) writes 'External feedback as a transmission

Pocket Guide to Teaching for Clinical Instructors, Third Edition.
Edited by Ian Bullock, Mike Davis, Andrew Lockey and Kevin Mackway-Jones.
© 2016 John Wiley & Sons, Ltd. Published 2016 by John Wiley & Sons, Ltd.

process involving "telling" ignores the active role the student must play in constructing meaning from feedback messages'.

The learning conversation

The learning conversation has two broad strands: first you need to elicit and explore issues that the learner identifies; after this you can raise issues that you noticed, but the learner did not mention and explore these. With both strands it is best if you can include the perceptions and perspectives of the rest of the group.

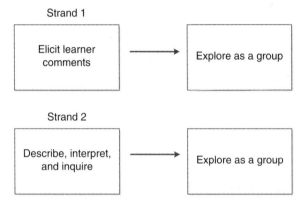

Figure 8.1 Overview of the learning conversation

It is best to consider this as a loose structure, for, as Carr (2006), writes:

> 'It is important that a variety of different techniques are used and that the approach be varied each time so the experience does not become predictable'.

Predictability has been raised as an issue by learners commenting on highly structured feedback they have received. In contrast a well-managed learning conversation leaves learners feeling relieved, valued and clear about their next steps. An approach that is genuinely conversational is not at risk of becoming predictable as it is responsive to the learner's agenda.

The learning conversation has been designed with tight time constraints in mind. When used effectively it is focussed, economical and supportive because of the lack of redundancy and a direct focus on issues raised by learners. It is shown in Box 8.1 and described in detail below:

Box 8.1 Feedback through dialogue

The Learning Conversation
- Starting the conversation
- Exploring any issues that emerge
- Exploring any issues that the learner identifies
- Including the group
- Sharing your thoughts
- Checking for unresolved issues
- Summarising

Starting the conversation

The facilitator should start the conversation by finding out what the learner wants to discuss. Sometimes this happens spontaneously. On other occasions learners wait for the instructor to initiate the conversation. In the latter case, this can be done in an open-ended or a focussed way with examples given below.

Box 8.2 Different approaches to starting the learning conversation

Open-ended
What did that simulation feel like?

Focussed
That's a difficult situation because of the complications introduced by the hypothermia, and you didn't get to that 'H' until the second cycle. Can you recall what prevented you from identifying the relevant reversible cause?

The open-ended approach allows the learner to choose what they want to talk about and this means that the issue that is uppermost in their minds can be dealt with. Often this is the one small error that they made in an otherwise good practice. On occasions they want to talk through the whole experience in order to make sense of it. Time constraints, however, emphasise the need to spotlight key aspects of the simulation and the focussed approach, as shown above, can be a convenient short cut for this.

Common errors at this stage
- Being long winded with your opening to the conversation
- Always using the same opening
- Delaying a topic introduced by the candidate in order to pursue your own agenda

Exploring the learner's issues

An exploration of the issue identified by the learner should follow seamlessly on from the start of the conversation. From the perspective of the facilitator, it will take the form either of silence or questions aimed at focussing on specific aspects of a performance. Learners have many ideas and profound insight if we give them time to formulate a thought. Many people learn through verbalising. If instructors verbalise for learners we deprive them of the possibility of being exploratory and of being reflective, hence the need to stop talking and leave spaces within the discussion. For the learning conversation to be effective, it needs to be responsive not pre-prepared and this means listening in a way that takes in all of the potential signals.

Occasionally facilitators suggest that learners defer issues so that they can be discussed later at the facilitator's discretion. Rudolph et al. (2007) show how dialogue structured by the facilitator in this way may create perceptions of inequality and lead to the facilitator dispensing wisdom to the hapless learner who is framed as the only person likely to be learning from the event. This is seductively easy as Hartwig et al. (1999) found.

It would have been easier for me to state and show 'this is the way to do it'.
I needed to be able to listen to and respond to the situation.

You may have observed facilitators making frequent use of examples from their own experience: comments such as 'When I get into that situation I find it useful to. . . .' This may be helpful to the learner but it is crucial not to overwhelm learners with your own personal experience when they are deep within the aftermath of the recent learning event. As a facilitator you need to spend more of your time listening than talking and this is often much more of a challenge than it sounds.

Effective listening occurs when the facilitator focusses on the learner with genuine interest without being distracted by working out what they are going to say next. It will also help if you are comfortable with silence and possess a non-hierarchical model of learning with a belief that others may have a perspective that will help enlighten the situation. Throughout the learning conversation, maintaining a global vigilance and processing non-verbal as well as verbal communication will give a wider channel of understanding.

Common errors at this stage
- Not listening and failing to pick up the learner's concerns
- Deferring issues: 'let's talk about that in a minute'
- Misinterpreting what the learner says
- Using pre-prepared phrases and disturbing the natural flow

Including the group

Low fidelity simulation is increasingly viewed as a group event with members of the group either being part of the team assisting during the simulation or observing. The feedback can, and should, involve the group in sharing their perspective on any issues that emerge. Consider the following diagrams in which the facilitator is marked in red, the team leader in black and the other group members in blue.

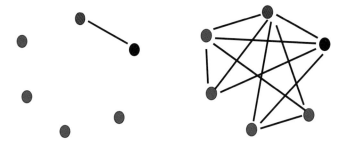

Figure 8.2 Facilitation styles during feedback

The first shows what has been described as 'verbal ping pong' (Askew and Lodge, 2000) between the facilitator and the learner. Feedback often takes this form. The second shows the conversation as a web. In this second example, the conversation sometimes goes through the facilitator but not always; the facilitator is vigilant but not dominant, has control but is not controlling. This is what we are aiming for with the learning conversation.

Perhaps the best way to ensure group involvement is to resist responding to the learner yourself. This strategy is explored in more detail in the chapter on facilitating small groups. You do not need to look disinterested, merely to leave spaces. You can also include the group by asking questions of individuals or of everyone. Examples are given below.

> **Examples of ways of involving the group**
> • What did anyone see to be the main issue with this patient?
> • [to the team] How did you see your role in the simulation?
> • How do you make sure you remember the drug doses?
> • What alternatives can anyone suggest for that difficult situation?

What we should avoid doing is asking the group to give the learner difficult feedback that we don't want to give ourselves. When the learner does need to be told about significant problems we should do that and in the next section we will suggest how best to do this.

> **Common errors at this stage**
> • Forgetting to include the group
> • Providing solutions yourself rather than using the resources within the group

Sharing your thoughts

In some settings, feedback is only allocated a few minutes, and in order to meet this time challenge, it is important not to waste time by reiterating comments that have already been made. Not only is this unnecessary but it undermines the discussion that has just happened. Equally you do not have time to list the learner's achievements, even though you may want to raise their esteem. It is more effective to highlight one or two key points as strengths or improvements.

When the facilitator is aware of an issue that has not been discussed, they are faced with the challenge of how to raise the issue in a way that encourages learning rather than defensiveness. The approach used increasingly in simulation centres is **advocacy with inquiry** which has its origins in action science (Argyris et al., 1985). It has come to the attention of practitioners of low and high fidelity simulation through the process described as 'Debriefing with good judgement' – see for example Rudolph et al. (2007) and the learning conversation used on life support courses throughout the world. Broadly speaking, when you want to raise a point for discussion you should provide the data (i.e. describe what you have noticed, being as specific as your recall allows), give your interpretation of this and then seek clarification from the learner about their perspective, or give them the opportunity to give their rationale for acting as they did.

Productive advocacy is descriptive and based on the specific data of the simulation rather than general and should have a non-judgemental quality to it (Chowdhury and Kalu, 2006). An example of judgemental, rather than descriptive feedback would be: 'You have a bit of a tendency to throw orders into the air and hope that someone will catch them'.

Certain phrases telegraph generic comments which are by their nature judgemental rather than descriptive: 'a bit of a tendency to … ' is one. Examples of others are

- you always …
- why don't you just …
- you don't seem to realise that …

For this issue to be raised in a beneficial way it would need to describe the behaviour. For example 'When you were checking the circulation you asked for a blood pressure reading and for the monitors to be put on'.

It can then be helpful, as indicated above, to acknowledge that you (the observer) have a perspective on this. For example *'I wasn't sure who this was directed at'*.

Having made your own thought process visible, it is possible to ask the learner to explore their thought processes. For example *'Can you recall what was going on from your perspective at that moment?'*

In this example, the facilitator's comment is firmly grounded in the data and this is the element that is often missing as facilitators try to get learners to work out for themselves what the problem is in a mistaken belief that this is an important part of the learning process. It is more effective to tell the learner what we consider to be the problem and encourage them to explore their actions and, if appropriate, identify alternative behaviour. They are then more likely to retain the knowledge having played a full part in the discussion and the solution.

Advocacy with inquiry is sometimes described in rather rigid terms but in reality, and in order to sound natural, it takes many forms. Some examples showing different approaches are given below.

A range of ways of raising difficult issues
- At that point I thought X was going on, *what did you think was happening?*
- When the patient collapsed it took you 2 minutes to initiate CPR and I was starting to get worried. *What was going through your mind at the time?*

> - I am wondering if … *does this sound like a possibility?*
> - I noticed that you put the oxygen on during your assessment of circulation; *can you tell me what prompted you to do that?*
> - During the simulation I gave you a bit of a hint about glucose and you looked frustrated with yourself that you'd forgotten it. *What are your thoughts on strategies for remembering it in future?*

When giving the learner feedback it may be helpful to think in the following terms:
- What did I see? (and give a description of this, being as accurate as possible)
- How did I interpret this? (acknowledge I have a perspective)
- Am I missing something? (be open to a range of responses rather than anticipating just one)

The moment the facilitator stops trying to force the learner into their frame and is interested in the learner's frame, acknowledging their constraints as real, it becomes possible for learning and change to occur. Constraints are usually tacit and unless they are consciously explored there is the risk that people's actions and behaviours will be misinterpreted.

> **Indicators of learners' constraints**
> - I didn't realise I was allowed to …
> - I thought we were supposed to …
> - I thought because it was a role-play it was okay to …
> - I was worried about …
> - I decided that on balance it would be better if I …
> - I did think about that, but the problem was …

Learners are vulnerable during feedback sessions, sometimes unwilling to enter into a prolonged conversation. They risk being given a lot of negative information as it is often easy on the outside to see a host of errors. Facilitators who are aware of this use empathy, distinct from pity or sympathy, to acknowledge that the situation the learner is in might be difficult, stressful and embarrassing. If the facilitator can have some level of emotional resonance with the learner, this understanding will enhance the learning process. Empathy may also mean deciding to withhold or defer some of the feedback.

A question we might usefully ask ourselves is: how do we find that which is genuinely positive when a scenario has not gone well? There are two issues here: the first is about maintaining our integrity, as learners find it hard to continue to trust an instructor who has been less than truthful because of a desire to remain positive. And the second is that we must ensure that learning occurs, that errors are corrected and that the learner is in a frame of mind to be able to listen, evaluate, interact and suggest alternative strategies.

There are a number of ways in which it is possible to be positive while remaining credible, honest and empathic.

1. Be positive about the learning that can occur.
2. Acknowledge how the learner must be feeling and their desire to improve.
3. Praise helpful suggestions for improvement and the learner's own perception of errors.
4. Listen attentively to the learners, support them and show that you value their personal reflections.
5. Focus on issues and solving puzzles rather than positives and negatives.

Common errors at this stage
- Listing good or bad points
- Returning to points that have already been discussed
- Using leading questions to mask your agenda
- Not using the data to inform your observations

Checking for unresolved issues and summarising

As you move towards the end of the learning conversation, check whether anyone has anything else that they would quickly like to discuss. Include within your sweep the team leader, the rest of the group and the other instructor in the room. The intention at this stage is simply to provide an opportunity to deal with any unresolved issues. Occasionally the candidates will make positive comments to the team leader which may indicate that the conversation has had a rather negative tone. As was discussed in the last section we must remain mindful of this.

Keep your summary brief as you will be repeating points that were only made a very short time ago. The purpose is to sum up the discussion in a succinct manner, highlighting achievable outcomes which should already have emerged. Some instructors like to ask the team leader to make their own summary and if this feels appropriate there is no harm in taking this approach. As with everything that we have discussed about the learning conversation it is important not to be overly rigid, but to keep the tone discursive rather than didactic, focussed on learning rather than teaching.

> **Common errors at this stage**
> * Asking the candidate if there is anything they would do differently: this has already been discussed.
> * Second instructor revisiting what has been said: they should only occasionally add anything.

Summary and learning

Feedback is one of the most valuable aspects of any teaching and learning event where practical situations and role-plays are encountered. In order to facilitate an effective learning conversation, the facilitator should maintain their credibility with the group, through listening and encouraging the group to share their perspectives to help solve any puzzles that emerge. Facilitators should also be willing to share their own perspective using the data rather than leading questions, and be honest, helpful and concrete in the feedback that they give, engaging in an informative and relevant dialogue with the learners.

References

Argyris C, Putnam R, Smith D. *Action Science*. Jossey-Bass, San Francisco, CA, 1985.

Askew S, Lodge C. Gifts, ping-pong and loops – linking feedback and learning. In: Askew S, ed. *Feedback for Learning*. Routledge, London, 2000; pp. 1–17.

Carr S. The foundation programme assessment tools: an opportunity to enhance feedback to trainees? *Postgraduate Medical Journal*, 2006;82:576–579.

Chowdhury R, Kalu G. Learning to give feedback in medical education. *Obstetrician and Gynaecologist*, 2006;6:243–247.

Hartwig K, Peach D, Taylor P. The reflective practitioner and the professional doctorate. *Changing Practice Through Research*, 1999;127–138.

Juwah C, McFarlane-Dick D, Matthew R, Nicol D, Ross D, Smith B. *Enhancing Student Learning Through Effective Formative Feedback*. The Higher Education Academy Generic Centre, 2004.

Pendleton D, Scofield T, Tate P, Havelock P. *The Consultation: An Approach to Learning and Teaching*. Oxford University Press, Oxford, 1984.

Rudolph J, Simon R, Rivard P, Dufresne R, Raemer D. Debriefing with Good Judgment: combining rigorous feedback with genuine inquiry. *Anaesthesiology Clinics*, 2007;25:361–376.

Saunders S and Gowing R. Learning from the learning conversation: benefits and problems in developing a process to improve workplace performance. In: Summary of Presentation at the 3rd International Conference 'Researching Vocational Education and Training'. 14–16 July 1999, Bolton Institute.

CHAPTER 9
e-Learning

Learning outcomes

By the end of this chapter you should be able to demonstrate an understanding of
* the nature of the e-learning experience from the point of view of the learner
* an approach to the development of online teaching materials

Introduction

e-Learning has had a surprisingly long history: it is over 40 years since computers first made their presence felt in higher education and almost 20 years since dedicated computer platforms, subsequently called virtual learning environments (VLEs), first appeared. Providers and funders of training across the world are beginning to accept the emerging importance of e-learning. Sensing this shift, many providers of continuing medical education have adopted a blended approach to some of their courses, combining the benefits of e-learning materials and traditional face-to-face (f2f) teaching.

Other, more contemporary, developments include the availability of apps for tablets and smart phones and the potential of social media for instructional and discussion purposes. For the purposes of this chapter, e-learning will include all kinds of e-learning (e.g. including m-learning – i.e. learning that makes use of mobile devices). Detailed attention, however, will not be paid to the most recent developments as this is such a rapidly expanding domain.

Pocket Guide to Teaching for Clinical Instructors, Third Edition.
Edited by Ian Bullock, Mike Davis, Andrew Lockey and Kevin Mackway-Jones.
© 2016 John Wiley & Sons, Ltd. Published 2016 by John Wiley & Sons, Ltd.

Regardless of the particular technology, e-learning has some characteristics, and in this chapter, we will explore these from a number of perspectives.

Background

Initially institutions (mis)used the Internet by the wholesale transfer of f2f courses from the conventional classroom to the virtual classroom, without taking the change in pedagogy into account. The inevitable outcome of this is that the worst features of the conventional classroom (i.e. a non-interactive lecture) are transplanted onto a computer screen. Thus, the learner's role is translated from passive listening in a lecture theatre to passive reading at a computer.

This situation began to change because of the influence of a number of educational technologists during the late 1990s. In more recent VLEs, learners are able to engage with materials in a more dynamic way through the use of a number of key characteristics:

- text (including interactive elements)
- images
- hyperlinks to other websites, including audio and video clips
- (reusable) learning objects
- person-to-person interaction

We will be exploring these in the following pages.

The advantages of e-learning

Text, figures and tables

Self-evidently, while text is still the dominant medium, online discourse has developed some of its own characteristics. This leads to a slightly less formal language and a more direct (to the reader) approach than, for example a textbook. Accordingly pages (screens) have fewer words and more illustrations and because the capacity exists, include interactive activities that engage the reader in a variety of ways. The range of interaction can be hinted at by consideration of this arm of a mind map produced to explore the notion of 'The ideal VLE' topic (Figure 9.1).

Tables and figures are readily embedded (i.e. as integral components of the online content) or can be accessed via links to web pages, for example www.gic-online.org/vle is the front page of the Generic Instructor Course VLE that some of you will have accessed.

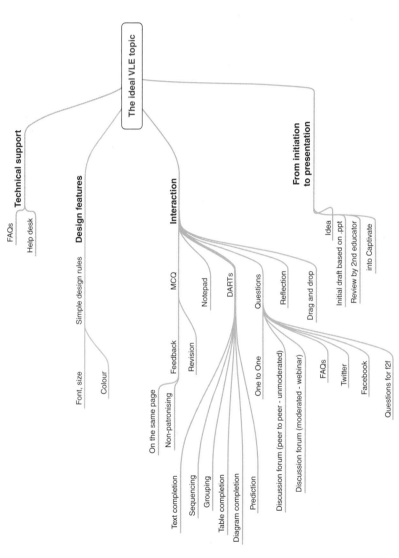

Figure 9.1 Extract from The Ideal VLE Topic

Other hyperlinks, including reusable learning objects

These can include websites, discussion areas, live feeds (e.g. RSS), podcasts and other audio and video material.

In some respects, all of the external links to the core text are what have come to be known as reusable learning objects. They are reusable in that they can be used in a wide variety of contexts, so have generic qualities and can also be accessed by any number of students in their original state. They can range from simple matching, pairing and prioritising activities to more complex animated teaching and learning tasks involving the virtual entry into a simulated environment.

In addition to these animated sites, the use of video and audio clips can add to the richness and complexity of the material. As an example, the medium of a videoed case conference or a disclosure interview in a child protection course can add considerably to the text.

Person-to-person interaction

Among the capabilities of online learning is the creation of interactive spaces and these can be either synchronous or asynchronous.

	Same time	Different time
Same place	Face-to-face meeting	Asynchronous conference; notice board; poster display
Different place	Synchronous conference; webinar, Twitter	Asynchronous conference, Twitter (plus summary content like "Storify")

In traditional VLEs, these can appear as forums or blogs and can be moderated or unmoderated. The capacity exists for these groups to be generated and sustained using social media like Facebook, YouTube and Twitter.

Limitations of e-learning

Some teaching modalities do not lend themselves readily to online learning and adjustments to the process have to be made. Take, for example skills teaching. Conventionally, within many life support courses, the preferred method of teaching skills is the four-stage approach – all four stages taking place in a single session. However, an online approach to skills teaching might consist of video clips of stages 1 and 2 followed by reinforcement and practice in f2f sessions that follow. An advantage of this would be that the video could include close-up shots of the skill, interspersed with clinical information or contexts, diagrams, photographs, and so on, thereby integrating the knowledge component of the skills. Furthermore, online learners can play the video as many times as they want (both before and after the f2f session).

VLEs can therefore supplement rather than replace f2f activity, so while some aspects of f2f work cannot currently be easily replicated online – for example role-play, scenarios and skills teaching, others can, to a greater or lesser extent. However, the VLE can be useful for the transference of knowledge-based content and for discussions about case studies. Knowledge-based programmes, clinical case study programmes and diagnostic support systems provide medical trainees with important access to material through e-learning.

A blended approach

e-Learning is increasingly seen as a contributor to a more blended approach to the learning experience. Carefully constructed VLEs containing appropriate text and a range of supporting activities and materials can enrich an experience not always available from books or manuals (notwithstanding developments in the e-book format). The opportunity to provide just-in-time learning with all of the interactive potential offered by the Internet as an introduction to the more challenging f2f environment, where practical issues can be explored, is one that is being adopted by a range of organisations from universities to continuing medical education providers.

Summary and learning

e-Learning has grown rapidly. When done well it is a considerable addition to the educational experience, contributing not only reinforcement but also depth and a degree of student control.

CHAPTER 10

Supporting learning

Learning outcomes

By the end of this chapter you should be able to demonstrate an understanding of
- the essential qualities of an instructor
- mentoring within a course and beyond

Introduction

There are a number of reasons why individuals become instructors. It may be because they enjoy teaching or because they are actively involved in a speciality or job that has a teaching commitment. It may be that becoming an instructor is an integral part of their career plan. Whatever the reasons, the role is both rewarding and motivating. Most instructors find that combining the theory learnt on courses with practical experience helps increase or maintain their own motivation. Finally, many find that although the role of an instructor is demanding and there are a few extrinsic rewards, it is an enjoyable, sociable and worthwhile activity.

What makes a good instructor?

Good instructors have a strong foundation of knowledge and skill that allow them to become (or at least aspire to becoming) role models for learners. The building blocks for this have been described by Hesketh et al. (2001) and are shown in Figure 10.1.

Pocket Guide to Teaching for Clinical Instructors, Third Edition.
Edited by Ian Bullock, Mike Davis, Andrew Lockey and Kevin Mackway-Jones.
© 2016 John Wiley & Sons, Ltd. Published 2016 by John Wiley & Sons, Ltd.

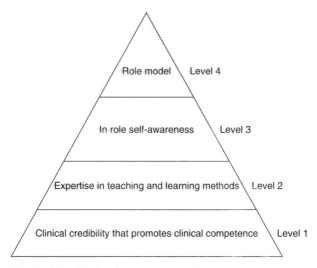

Figure 10.1 Building blocks of an instructor

Source: Hesketh 2001. Reprinted with permission of Wiley & Sons.

Level 1: clinical credibility

The foundations for instructor performance are the knowledge, skills and experience that each individual brings to their role. This means that the ability to teach includes an ability to demonstrate:

- clinical application of the theoretical content from the provider course
- understanding of the clinical context
- knowledge and credibility

Level 2: expertise in teaching and learning methods

A good instructor will make learning relevant, meaningful and fun, with all teaching sessions prepared thoroughly. Contrary to traditional approaches in healthcare and medical education, candidates will not simply consume what is read and said to them. Teaching is about providing the optimal conditions for effective learning, where candidates become active participants in the learning process. Key components for instructors to be able to achieve this are competency in teaching methods and understanding of how to facilitate candidate learning.

Level 3: in role self-awareness

'I want to change, but not if it means changing'—Grosz, 2014

Good instructors, by being aware of themselves and of their learners' needs and abilities, add a dynamic quality to the learning experience so that more than simple content is being covered. A key attribute is the ability to recognise the individual needs and strengths of each candidate. Understanding the principles outlined in this book, together with good interpersonal skills and a healthy attitude in the learning environment, should enable the instructor to provide feedback and support, enabling candidate growth and development. This will help them to overcome any barriers that they may have to learning from experience – something explored in Chapter 1.

Level 4: role model

Experienced instructors will tell you that they themselves learn something new from each course they attend. Their ability to reflect and learn in action (on the job) adds to their credibility as an instructor. Learning has been described as a journey not a destination.

Capturing this journey is encouraged and this can be achieved by maintaining a professional portfolio, where experiences gained can be maximised through reflection on practice.

Mentorship

Most courses require instructors to act as mentors to specific groups of candidates. Mentorship can be described as a relationship that fosters support in many areas including teaching, supervision, guidance, counselling, assessment and evaluation. It is clear that the instructor must remain focussed on the outcomes required from mentor/mentee meetings. These mentor meetings should be structured in such a way as to give time for group mentorship as well as the all-important individual mentorship. It is vital that candidates are given the opportunity to discuss their individual needs away from the group and that this is seen as being a programmed element and not only reserved for the struggling candidate.

The key role of the mentor is as teacher and critical friend. The teacher element is less distinct during time-limited mentor/mentee meetings. Mentors should be aware of who their specific group is and observe their development throughout the course, giving structured feedback when and where appropriate. This naturally leads to the critical friend role whereby mentors can give open and honest feedback having developed a level of rapport with their mentees.

Initial mentor meetings may not be very productive unless mentors have had contact with their mentees. This is where instructor responsibilities as a mentor become clear. The instructor who has to leave early or is late in arriving to the course will not be in a position to offer professional mentorship and risks losing credibility with mentees. A good course timetable will arrange for mentors to be grouped together having contact with their mentees at the beginning and end of each day and during informal contact, like refreshment breaks and lunchtime. In addition, important information about a candidate's performance may only become evident at the faculty meeting, after the course has dispersed for the day. Mentors must ensure that they feedback any relevant information to their mentees before commencement of the following day's course.

Other issues

Attending meetings

On many courses there are faculty meetings at the beginning of the course and at the end of each day. The initial meeting is a forum for all instructors to meet since often they may not know each other and have probably not all taught together before. The course director and the course co-ordinator can introduce instructors to each other, discuss the layout of the teaching environment, note any last minute changes to the programme and importantly, discuss the approach to any contentious areas that are being addressed.

The initial meeting also provides an opportunity to ensure that all instructors are prepared for the day ahead. Instructors teaching overlapping topics can use the opportunity to check which areas they are each covering and to ensure a consistent approach. Faculty meetings at the end of the day should be more focussed on the candidates themselves, although any logistical or controversial issues, which have arisen during the day, may be discussed and rectified. The main aim of the discussion about the candidates is to identify those who need remedial help and to formulate a plan to deliver this. The assessments, which are collated from any formative feedback sheets should be used to assist in this process.

At the final faculty meeting, any formative and summative assessments are discussed. On some courses, learners may pass, retest in a particular area or it may be recommended that they repeat the course in its entirety. Some participants may be offered the opportunity to teach.

Supporting other instructors

Occasionally, the instructor who is carrying out a session is less confident and may require both moral and practical support. Instructors must show support for instructors in this position both by being there (for instance, by sitting in at the back of the lecture room) and by stepping in to answer difficult questions raised by candidates if these occur.

Regulations and requirements

Course providers have similar regulations with regard to developing and maintaining instructor status, recertification and a code of conduct, and it is important to familiarise yourself with those that apply. Many governing bodies maintain central lists of all qualified instructors and these are made available to course centres to allow them to invite instructors. Instructors will also be sent lists of the course centres and course dates to allow them to approach suitable centres if they so wish.

Summary and learning

As an instructor, you will be part of a faculty of experienced people teaching knowledge and skills to adult learners. The instructor role is rewarding and demands highly motivated and reliable individuals who display knowledge and credibility in the field of resuscitation.

References

Grosz S. *The Examined Life*. Vintage Books, London, 2014.

Hesketh E, Bagnall G, Buckley E, Friedman M, Goodall M, Harden R, Laidlaw J, Leighton-Beck L, McKinley P, Newton R, Oughton R. A frame-work for developing excellence as a clinical educator. *Medical Education*, 2001;35(6):555–564.

CHAPTER 11
Teaching teams

Learning outcomes

By the end of this chapter you should be able to demonstrate
- an understanding of the key aspects of team leadership
- an appreciation of the key aspects of team working
- an understanding of how these skills, roles and functions can be facilitated through effective teaching

Introduction

Thousands of doctors, nurses and paramedics are now trained every year in adult, paediatric and neonatal emergency care, and the courses designed to train them have become embedded in profession-specific specialist training curricula. While the development of *the individual* in technical skills has been a real benefit from these courses, it has become apparent that all the courses need to develop a more *team-based* approach in line with increasing awareness of the role of non-technical skills.

The 'Clinical Human Factors Group' working definition of human factors is useful for providing both context and content for learning:

Human factors are all the things that make us different from logical, completely predictable machines. How we think and relate to other people, equipment and our environment. It is about how we perform in our roles and how we can optimise that performance to improve safety and efficiency. In simple terms it's the things that affect our personal performance.

Pocket Guide to Teaching for Clinical Instructors, Third Edition.
Edited by Ian Bullock, Mike Davis, Andrew Lockey and Kevin Mackway-Jones.
© 2016 John Wiley & Sons, Ltd. Published 2016 by John Wiley & Sons, Ltd.

Typically team members are aware of the focussed tasks they are responsible for, with the team leader trying to co-ordinate these aspects of technical care. In simulated settings, instructors quietly facilitate progress by feeding vital information to the team leader, who has to recognise life-threatening problems and address them. They must keep calm and use situation awareness (Reason, 2008) of deteriorating vital signs, risks with equipment and team member effectiveness, team dynamic and patient response to interventions. This is a highly complex context which demands high-level functioning at both a cognitive and behavioural level.

How can we teach teams to work together?

Fuhrmann et al. (2009) trained people in their own teams with good outcomes. Billington (2004) characterises much of what the resuscitation provider courses aim to achieve with regard to teaching non-technical skills, in three elements of team functioning. These are
• Commitment
• Competence
• Common goal
   Norris and Lockey (2010) added two further 'C's: communication and conflict management. Communication helps a team define their common goal and facilitates conflict resolution.
   In understanding how we as teachers can facilitate the development of team function using the simulated setting, we need to understand ways to increase the authenticity for the learner by emphasising the team common goal (which in healthcare should always be the best care of and outcome for the patient). Max Ringelmann quoted by Huczynski and Buchanan (2005) also gives helpful pointers to teachers, indicating that learners are motivated more effectively if the team leader
• knows the names of team members
• allocates roles to individuals that they perceive as important and which are appropriate to their experience
   Two aspects of performance can be enhanced by good simulation teaching. These are leadership and team dynamics. The two boxes below provide instructors with pointers to improving performance in these two areas.

Using teaching scenarios to augment both team leadership and team learning:
- Provide clinical information to the team leader
- Provide information to the wider team
- Enable situation awareness to develop
- Give positive feedback 'in scenario' that augments both individual and group learning

Using teaching scenarios to explore team dynamic and facilitate team learning:
- Emphasise that team members should be committed to a good patient outcome
- Encourage team members to communicate clearly
- Enable team members to support the team leader
- Engage all team members in the learning conversation to emphasise key points. If you ask a question and the team leader is slow answering, reflect the question to the team. This motivates the team members to listen to the scenario and aids teamwork as they have to help their team leader.
- Use a scribe (allocated team member) to be part of the iterative feedback and learning
- Involve the group members in the learning conversation to make suggestions for the team leader. This removes the 'spotlight' from the individual receiving feedback and encourages the bonding of the team and group reflection on their actions.

This approach allows for the situation learning of the team to be enhanced. By sharing the importance of these aspects of effective team function, teachers not only build confidence in the team but can also emphasise the team leader role, characteristics and behaviours which can then translate from a simulated to a clinical setting. The team leader needs to appraise team function, something which the teacher can again facilitate 'in scenario' by exploring how the team leader is functioning and by appraising team performance as well as patient response to interventions and outcome. Leadership traits and team function can be assessed by both the teacher and in peer settings, using the 'Team Emergency Assessment Measure (TEAM)' developed by Cooper et al. (2010). This provides opportunity for dynamic 'learning conversations' to shape both individual and team feedback. Good team leadership involves the attributes shown in the box:

> • Know their team members by name and have insight into their capability
> • Accept the leadership role
> • Are knowledgeable and have sufficient credibility to influence the team through role modelling and professionalism
> • Stay calm and enable the team to be focussed (Pardey 2004)
> • Are a good communicator (good listener and decisive in action)
> • Delegate tasks appropriately
> • Drive patient management in a time-sensitive environment and establish priorities
> • Demonstrate situation awareness (Reason 2008)

Summary and learning

Good team functioning has been demonstrated to have a positive effect on patient outcome. By developing an understanding of team behaviours as well as team leadership in resuscitation courses, we may enhance teamwork in patient settings and improve outcomes.

References

Billington J. *'Teams That click.* Harvard Business School Press, Boston, MA, 2004.

Cooper S, Cant R, Porter J, Sellick K, Somers G, Kinsmanc L, Nestel D. Rating medical emergency teamwork performance: development of the Team Emergency Assessment Measure (TEAM). *Resuscitation*, 2010;81:446–452.

Fuhrmann L, Østergaard D, Lippert A, Perner A. A multi-professional full scale simulation course in the recognition and management of deteriorating hospital patients. *Resuscitation*, 2009, 80(6):669–673.

Huczynski A, Buchanan D. *Organisational Behaviour – An Introductory Text*, 5th ed. Financial Times Prentice Hall, Harlow, Essex, 2005.

Norris EM, Lockey AS. Human factors and resuscitation teaching. *Resuscitation,* 2010;81(2):32–34.

Pardey D (2004) *'Leading teams'*, Institute of Leadership and Management, Stowe House, Staffs.

Reason J. *The Human Contribution. Unsafe Acts, Accidents and Heroic Recoveries.* Ashgate, Manchester, UK, 2008.

Index

Pocket Guide to Teaching for Clinical Instructors, Third Edition.
Edited by Ian Bullock, Mike Davis, Andrew Lockey and Kevin Mackway-Jones.
© 2016 John Wiley & Sons, Ltd. Published 2016 by John Wiley & Sons, Ltd.